One Path Among Many

One Path Among Many

a cancer patient's experiences and insights
about his personal journey

By Robert Koshinskie

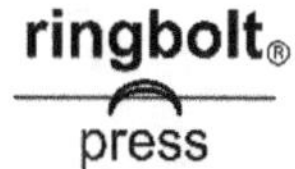

One Path Among Many

ISBN 9798837716065 (Paperback)

ASIN: B0BBD5ZVTG (eBook)

Publisher's Cataloging-in-Publication data

Names: Koshinskie, Robert, author.
Title: One path among many: a cancer patient's experiences
and insights about his personal journey / by Robert
Koshinskie.
Description: Includes bibliographical references. | Burlington,
NC: Robert Koshinskie as Ringbolt Press, 2022.
Identifiers: ISBN: 9798837716065 (paperback)
Subjects: LCSH Koshinskie, Robert--Health. | Cancer
patients--Biography. | Pancreas--Cancer--Patients. | BISAC
BIOGRAPHY & AUTOBIOGRAPHY / Personal Memoirs |
HEALTH & FITNESS / Diseases & Conditions / Cancer |
PHILOSOPHY / Mind & Body
Classification: LCC RC265.8.K67 2022 | DDC 616.99/092--
dc23

First edition 8 October 2022

Cover photograph by kinkate from Pixabay

Dedication

To all cancer patients, their families, and friends,

"Get busy with life's purpose, toss aside empty hopes, get active in your own rescue – if you care for yourself at all – and do it while you can."

– Marcus Aurelius,
Roman emperor and practitioner of Stoicism

TABLE OF CONTENTS

Acknowledgments

Diane Pinder, my wife, and Clinical Research Nurse Coordinator (CRNC) at Duke University Health System. I couldn't have asked for a more loving spouse or more skilled nurse advocate in my care. Diane's many years of experience at the bedside with patients and working with cancer researchers enable her to translate medical information for me, and to work closely with my health care team who coordinate my care plan. Diane also reviewed my drafts for this book and filled in the blanks that my "chemo brain" did not properly recall.

Hope E. Uronis, MD, Margot Mahon O'Neill, PA, Rebecca Ann Burbridge, MD, all the other members of my Duke oncology health care team, and all the employees that I interact with during my visits at Duke Hospital. I appreciate your professionalism, skill, and empathy.

Steven Merlin, a ten-year pancreatic cancer survivor who has experienced cancer therapies from the Whipple surgical procedure[1] to a clinical trial for targeted therapy that resulted in achieving no evidence of disease (NED) in Steven as of April 2016.[2] Steven's professional career spans 35 years in academic and government research labs and the life sciences industry. Initially trained as a Medical Technologist, Steven has worked at the National Institute of Allergy and Infectious Diseases (NIAID) and the National Heart, Lung, and Blood Institute (NHLBI), the University of Bern, the Ludwig Institute for Cancer Research, Columbia University College of Physicians and Surgeons, and the Weill Cornell Medical College. Steven currently serves as the Outreach Chair for the NJ affiliate of the Pancreatic Cancer Action Network. Steven was very gracious with his time, speaking with Diane and me, reviewing and commenting on my book draft, and providing the Foreword for this book. I've included several of Steven's insightful comments verbatim in the body of this book with attribution.

Tom and Lynne Hogan are both old friends from college. Tom's experience as a Chief Financial Officer, and General Manager affords him an eye for detail. His witty and blunt critiques of my drafts helped me craft a straightforward, plain English narrative. Tom's wife Lynne is a two-time breast cancer survivor who graciously reviewed my drafts and shared her own experiences and thoughts with me.

Foreword

In 2012 when I was diagnosed with pancreatic cancer, I found myself facing a catastrophic illness and needing to find relevant information so I could make informed decisions. My searches focused on finding scientific papers documenting patient case histories resulting in survival. Working in the field of medical research in cancer and immunology, I had familiarity with terminology and statistics. But this did not fully meet my needs for practical information to deal with this disease on a daily basis.

This recalcitrant cancer is treatable and survivable but requires dealing with adversity, remaining undaunted, and having perseverance. One will encounter emotional, mental, physical, and spiritual challenges. What would have been helpful to me as a patient and those that served as caregivers was a publication written from the patient perspective where all the information was clear, concise, and organized. Over the years I have read many patient blogs but found it required time-consuming searches for specific information. When Robert contacted me explaining his project, it sounded like what I had been searching for so long.

Like a handy travel guide that orients the reader to a foreign land and culture, this book is a useful tool to help cancer patients and their families navigate their own paths. *One Path Among Many* is a first-hand, practical account of what a patient will likely experience on their cancer journey with valuable suggestions, tips, and sources for finding specific information.

Steven Merlin
Outreach Chair for the New Jersey affiliate of the Pancreatic Cancer Action Network

Preface

By nature, I'm a private person who is somewhat *emotionally closed*. I was raised in an environment at a time that promoted independence and dealing with one's problems without complaining. Boys learned from an early age that it wasn't *manly* or acceptable to show emotion or ask for help. Corporal punishment was an accepted method of corrective discipline in those days.

For the reasons above and others, the idea of sharing my personal cancer journey put me on unsteady ground. How much was I willing to expose myself in ways I hadn't done before? After some reflection, I decided that if I could help others, even in some small way, then revealing myself was a trivial price to pay.

My purpose in writing this book is to share my experiences as a pancreatic cancer patient. I hope to provide some clear-eyed perspective and useful insight to newly diagnosed cancer patients, their families, and friends.

This book is about moving forward daily by identifying and acting on the few things we can control in our lives and identifying and accepting the many things over which we have no control. This approach may seem common sense on its face but doing so can be challenging to many and completely unacceptable to others.

Everyone has one life to live on their own terms and everyone will follow their own path among the many paths that others pursue. I'm not trying to convert you to my way of thinking, and I make no claim that my approach is the "right" way for you.

Whatever path you choose, I wish you and yours the best on your journey.

Robert Koshinskie

Introduction

2022 started out in sorrow with the deaths of my wife Diane's parents – her father passed on New Year's Day and her mother a week later. Diane's parents had been ill for some years and Diane was their active advocate, managing their many and challenging medical and personal affairs. It was a grueling time for Diane, and it looked like things would be better in the New Year.

At the beginning of 2022, I was a product owner for the development of a novel hospital bedside patient monitor and central station system. It was an ambitious and stimulating project, located squarely in my medical device "sweet spot" and I was working with an experienced and skilled team. I also started the year with my annual wellness check that indicated I was in good health.

Diane was employed as a clinical research nurse coordinator (CRNC) at Duke University Health System. In her role, she ensured that cancer studies were moving forward smoothly, coordinating the needs of researchers and patients alike. Before my diagnosis, I had a vague understanding of Diane's responsibilities, but I didn't realize the vital part that Diane's expertise would soon play in our lives.

In a couple of years preceding my diagnosis Diane and I had fashioned a retirement plan that would lead us from full-time employment to part-time employment to volunteer work. We would each spend time on our interests like Diane's painting and my recent exploration of Japanese woodworking. We would travel to places in the States that we had discussed over the years and return to the Tuscany area in Italy that we had enjoyed years earlier. In short, smooth sailing ahead for 2022 and beyond. But everything started to change just weeks into the new year.

In February of 2022, I started experiencing significant abdominal pain after eating that radiated into my chest and back. Initially diagnosed as a common gastrointestinal issue that more fiber and water would resolve, it turned out that I had a malignant tumor on my pancreas. Our hopes for a better year and a simple life in retirement quickly faded. As boxer Mike

Tyson has opined, "Everybody has a plan until they get punched in the mouth."

Faced with a serious cancer diagnosis our lives changed overnight. I canceled my work contract to focus on my treatment. Diane took on the added role of my nurse-advocate, coordinating a care plan for me. Very quickly, our lives became all about hospital appointments and dealing with the effects of my disease and treatment. I was experiencing Diane's expertise and her amazing ability to take control of an urgent medical situation firsthand.

I am very fortunate to be living near a major oncology center and to have a wife who is also an ideal nurse-advocate. However, actually living with the disease rather than being an observer raised many questions and issues that Diane and I never considered before. We wondered what lies ahead and if we have what it takes to roll with the jabs, hooks, and undercuts that cancer and cancer therapy throws.

This book – part explanation and part meditation, is for the recently diagnosed cancer patient, family, and friends. Although everyone's cancer journey is different, there are some common themes and information that may help the reader navigate the weeks and months ahead. The layout of this book is as follows.

- A very basic overview of cancer in general and pancreatic cancer, in particular, to help ensure the reader has a rudimentary understanding of key points
- A review of the procedures that I've undergone and to which I'll refer in my personal story
- My personal cancer story from the first signs of trouble, to diagnosis, to the therapy I'm receiving, and some bumps in the road along the way
- My experience with patient portals and planning documents – important tools that I strongly recommend you embrace
- My thoughts on emotional, religious, and philosophical issues – common in life-and-death situations, my views also create a foundation for the final section of the book
- How I'm working to maintain a healthy perspective and how I'm *dealing* with my disease and prognosis

The *explanation* parts of this book include the nuts-and-bolts factual descriptions, primarily in the sections: Cancer in General, Procedures, and much of the Appendices.

The *meditation* parts include my perspectives and thoughts, primarily in the sections: My Cancer Journey, Emotional, Religious and Philosophical Perspectives, and Wrapping it Up.

***

> I format information that I want to draw your attention to using an indent and a black border like this paragraph and the ones below. This information may include suggestions, clarifications, meditations, and such.

> I urge you to follow the numerous endnotes that I've provided (the little superscript numbers like [45] that appear next to quotes and claims). I supplied these references so you can read my sources of information and learn more at your convenience.

> I also urge you to read the Appendices where I offer a variety of information that I hope is useful and handy to you, your family, and friends.

> I use the pronouns and adjectives *he, him, his, she, her, and hers* randomly throughout this book as the traditional way to include all readers. The use of these terms is not intended to offend or exclude those in the LGBTQ+ community or any other reader.[3] Pancreatic cancer treats everyone with disrespect, regardless of their sex, gender, age, faith, or politics. We're all in this together.

> If you find this book to be a useful reference for yourself or others, then please help spread the word.

CANCER IN GENERAL & PANCREATIC CANCER IN PARTICULAR

Note that I do not claim any medical expertise. Much of the technical information contained in this book has been gathered from reputable sources but **none of it is intended as medical advice.**

I urge you to refrain from using "Dr. Google" where you will doubtless find unreliable and misleading information.

Look to websites that end in ".org", ".edu", and ".gov" that generally contain factual information, some of which is peer-reviewed or screened by an editor.

Always discuss your health and therapy, including anything you find on the Internet, with your health care team who can authoritatively answer your questions in detail.

What is Cancer?

Before I got my cancer diagnosis, I thought I knew what cancer *was*. The more I read about cancer, however, the more I realized how little I actually understood about the disease. So, let's start with a brief overview of cancer in general and how pancreatic cancer is different from other cancers. According to the National Cancer Institute (bold is mine):[4]

- Cancer is a disease in which some of the body's **cells grow uncontrollably and spread to other parts of the body.**
- **There are more than 100 types of cancer.** Types of cancer are usually named for the organs or tissues where the cancers form. For example, lung cancer starts in the lung, and brain cancer starts in the brain. Cancers also may be described by the type of cell that formed them, such as an epithelial cell or a squamous cell.

- **Cancer can start almost anywhere in the human body**, which is made up of trillions of cells. Normally, human cells grow and multiply (through a process called cell division) to form new cells as the body needs them. When cells grow old or become damaged, they die, and new cells take their place.

- **Sometimes this orderly process breaks down, and abnormal or damaged cells grow and multiply when they shouldn't.** These cells may form tumors, which are lumps of tissue. Tumors can be cancerous or not cancerous (benign).

- **Cancerous tumors spread into, or invade, nearby tissues and can travel to distant places in the body to form new tumors** (a process called metastasis). Cancerous tumors may also be called malignant tumors. Many cancers form solid tumors, but cancers of the blood, such as leukemias, generally do not.

- Benign tumors do not spread into, or invade, nearby tissues. When removed, **benign tumors usually don't grow back, whereas cancerous tumors sometimes do.** Benign tumors can sometimes be quite large, however. Some can cause serious symptoms or be life-threatening, such as benign tumors in the brain.

- Cancer is a genetic disease – that is, **it is caused by changes to genes that control the way our cells function, especially how they grow and divide.**

- The body normally eliminates cells with damaged DNA before they turn cancerous. **But the body's ability to do so goes down as we age.** This is part of the reason why there is a higher risk of cancer later in life.

- Each person's cancer has a unique combination of genetic changes. **As the cancer continues to grow, additional changes will occur.** Even within the same tumor, different cells may have different genetic changes.

- **A cancer that has spread from the place where it first formed to another place in the body is called metastatic cancer.** The process by which cancer cells spread to other parts of the body is called metastasis.

- **Metastatic cancer has the same name and the same type of cancer cells as the original, or primary, cancer.** For example, breast cancer that forms a metastatic tumor in the lung is metastatic breast cancer, not lung cancer.

What Causes Cancer?

Medical science is learning more about cancer every day and certain factors have been associated with cancer. According to Stanford Healthcare[5], however, (bold is mine):

- **There is no one single cause for cancer.** Scientists believe that it is the interaction of many factors together that produces cancer. The factors involved may be genetic, environmental, or constitutional characteristics of the individual.
- As mentioned, some cancers, particularly in adults, have been associated with repetitive exposures or risk factors. A risk factor is anything that may increase a person's chance of developing a disease. A risk factor does not necessarily cause the disease, but it may make the body less resistant to it. The following risk factors and mechanisms have been proposed as contributing to cancer:
  - **Lifestyle factors.** Smoking, a high-fat diet, and working with toxic chemicals are examples of lifestyle choices that may be risk factors for some adult cancers.
  - **Family history,** inheritance, and genetics may play an important role in some childhood cancers. It is possible for cancer of varying forms to be present more than once in a family. It is unknown in these circumstances if the disease is caused by a genetic mutation, exposure to chemicals near a family's residence, a combination of these factors, or simply coincidence.
  - **Environmental exposures.** Pesticides, fertilizers, and power lines have been researched for a direct link to childhood cancers. There has been evidence of cancer occurring among nonrelated children in certain neighborhoods and/or cities. Whether prenatal or infant exposure to these agents causes cancer, or whether it is a coincidence, is unknown.
  - **Some forms of high-dose chemotherapy and radiation.** In some cases, children who have been exposed to these agents may develop a second malignancy later in life. These strong anticancer agents can alter cells and/or the immune system. A second malignancy is a cancer that appears as a result from treatment of a different cancer.

What is Pancreatic Cancer?

As noted above, pancreatic cancer is cancer that originates in the pancreas. If pancreatic cancer spreads or grows to other organs like the liver (*metastasizes*), then it is referred to as pancreatic rather than liver cancer. So, what is the pancreas and how does it normally work in conjunction with the liver?

Let's start by looking at the first illustration below that shows the liver beneath our lungs and the pancreas sitting beneath our liver. In the second illustration, you can see that both the pancreas and liver are connected to the intestines via a series of tubes that carry the secretion of a gland (*ducts*). Further, the pancreas has three zones: head, body, and tail.

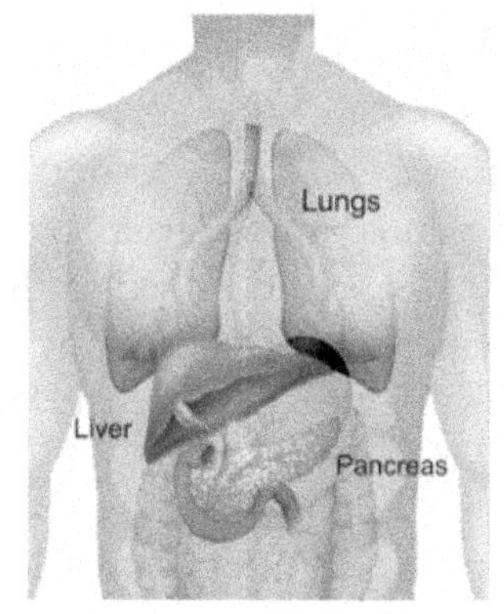

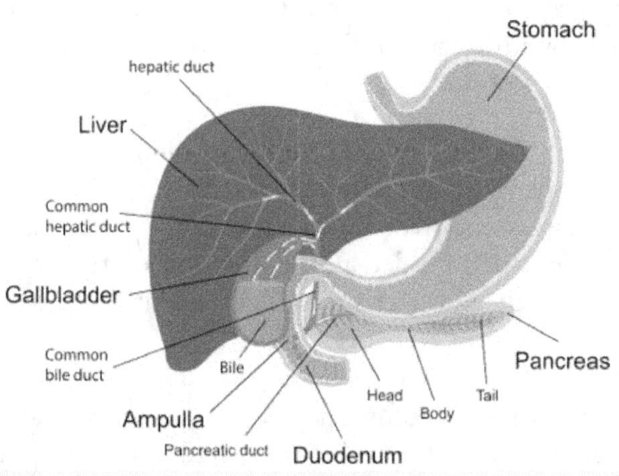

The pancreas is composed of cells that produce and transport enzymes which are released into ducts and then passed into the duodenum (the first part of the small bowel), where they aid in the digestion of food. The pancreas also has components within its cells that release hormones such as insulin and glucagon into the bloodstream. Insulin and glucagon maintain the proper level of sugar (*glucose*) in the blood, and blood sugar is used by our body for energy.[6]

The pancreatic duct combines with the bile duct and this short segment referred to as the common bile duct (CBD) connects to a segment small intestine known as the duodenum where pancreatic juice (mixture of digestive enzymes) enters. The *duodenum* is "the first and shortest section of the small intestine, is a key organ in the digestive system. The small intestine's most important function is to digest nutrients and pass them into the blood vessels – located in the intestinal wall – for absorption of the nutrients into the bloodstream."[7]

Note, too, the green *gallbladder* that connects ducts from the liver which also empty into the duodenum. These ducts carry *bile*, "a fluid that is made and released by the liver and stored in the gallbladder. Bile helps with digestion. It emulsifies fats by breaking large fat globules into smaller emulsion droplets increasing the surface area for the lipase enzyme to digest fats faster.[8]

The liver also clears a component called *bilirubin* which can accumulate and turn the skin and eyes yellow. When the liver has broken down harmful substances, its by-products are excreted into the bile or blood. Bile by-products enter the intestine and leave the body in the form of feces. Blood by-products are filtered out by the kidneys and leave the body in the form of urine.[9]

Now that you have a general understanding of the location and function of the pancreas and liver, you can see why any disease that impacts the pancreas and liver can significantly interfere with our body's ability to provide much-needed nutrients. One of the consequences of insufficient pancreatic and liver function is weight loss. According to the Pancreatic Cancer Action Network:

> "Weight loss is a common problem in individuals with pancreatic cancer. It can be associated with treatment or with the cancer itself. Tumor-induced weight loss, also

known as *cancer cachexia*, is a complex problem. It affects the way the body uses calories and protein. Cancer cachexia can cause the body to burn more calories than usual, break down muscle protein and decrease appetite. If a person is consuming regular meals and snacks but is losing weight, they may be experiencing cancer cachexia."[10]

Pancreatic Cancer by the Numbers

Although relatively rare, pancreatic cancer is known by the general public, in part, to a list of celebrities who had the disease, such as:

- Game show host Alex Trebek
- Actress Joan Crawford
- Actor John Hurt
- Actor Alan Rickman
- Astronaut Sally Ride
- Supreme Court Justice Ruth Bader Ginsburg
- Entrepreneur Steve Jobs
- Singer Aretha Franklin
- Singer Luciano Pavarotti
- Musician Dizzy Gillespie
- Actor Patrick Swayze
- Athlete Gene Upshaw

The graph below is from the National Cancer Institute (NCI)[11] and provides a summary of estimated new cases of pancreatic cancer shown as light green boxes [ ] and deaths shown as downward dark green triangles [▼] for 2022, and the 5-year survival rate.

Note that the annual number of new pancreatic cancer as a proportion of the number of people at risk for the disease (*incidence rate*) is 3.2% of all new cancer cases. However, pancreatic cancer accounts for 8.2 % of all cancer deaths. According to the Hirshberg Foundation for Pancreatic Cancer Research, "Pancreatic cancer has the highest mortality rate of all major cancers. It is currently the 3rd leading cause of cancer-related death in the United States after lung and colon and is expected to become the 2nd by 2030."[12]

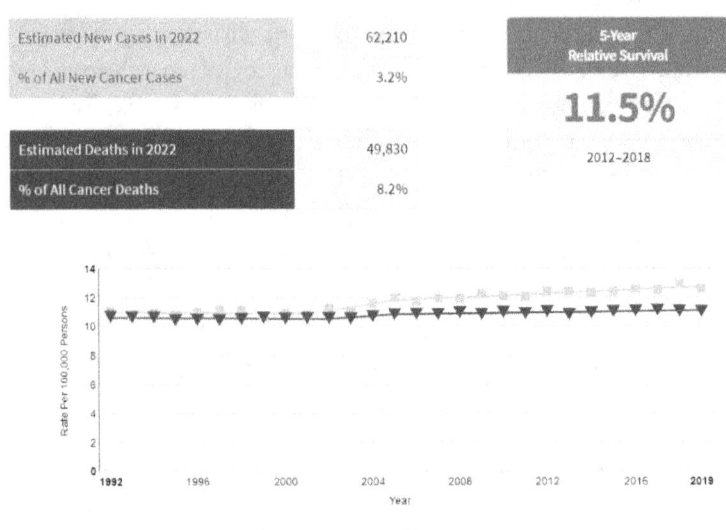

Cancers grow through stages, starting in an organ like the pancreas and then appearing in other organs like the liver and lung. Cancers may be designated by Stage (I-IV) or by the National Cancer Institute (NCI) Surveillance, Epidemiology, and End Results (SEER) Program survival categories:

- **Localized**: There is no sign that the cancer has spread outside of the pancreas.
- **Regional**: The cancer has spread from the pancreas to nearby structures or lymph nodes.
- **Distant**: The cancer has spread to distant parts of the body such as the lungs, liver, or bones.

The table below is based on people diagnosed with pancreatic cancer between 2011 and 2017.

SEER Stage	5-Year Relative Survival Rate
Localized	42%
Regional	14%
Distant	3%
All SEER Stages Combined	11%

Because staging may be confusing to the reader who has no medical expertise, the American Cancer Society advises[13] that (bold is mine),

- **These numbers apply only to the stage of the cancer when it is first diagnosed**. They do not apply later on if the cancer grows, spreads, or comes back after treatment.
- **These numbers don't take everything into account**. Survival rates are grouped based on how far the cancer has spread, but your age, overall health, how well the cancer responds to treatment, tumor grade, extent of resection, level of tumor marker (CA 19-9), and other factors will also affect your outlook.
- **People now being diagnosed with pancreatic cancer may have a better outlook than these numbers show**. Treatments improve over time, and these numbers are based on people who were diagnosed and treated at least five years earlier.

If one is fortunate enough to catch pancreatic cancer in its earliest stages, then they may benefit from a special operation, the Whipple procedure. According to the Mayo Clinic, "Your chances of long-term survival after a Whipple procedure depend on your particular situation. For most tumors and cancers of the pancreas, the Whipple procedure is the only known cure."[14] Due to the normally late detection and effectiveness of current pancreatic cancer therapies, however, the course and likely outcome of pancreatic cancer (*prognosis*) are frankly bleak.[15] Consider the *Long-Term Trends in SEER Age-Adjusted Incidence Rates* graph below.[16]

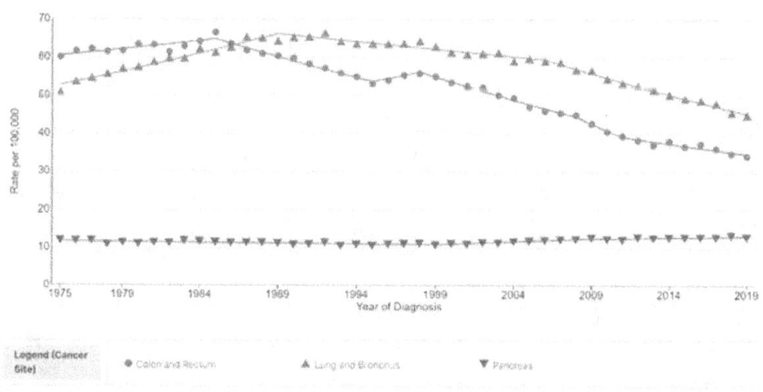

The graph above includes both male and female subjects, of all races and of all ages. The red circles [●] represent cancer of the colon and rectum, the blue upward triangles [▲] represent cancer of the lung and bronchus, and the green downward triangles [▼] represent cancer of the pancreas. It's plain that the incidence rate of pancreatic cancer is low, and when compared to other cancers its incidence rate is not improving.

Take a look at the *SEER 5-Year Relative Survival Rates* graph[17] below and you can see that survival rates for cancers of the colon and rectum (left red bar) and lung and bronchus (middle blue bar) are both higher than the survival rate for cancer of the pancreas (right green bar).

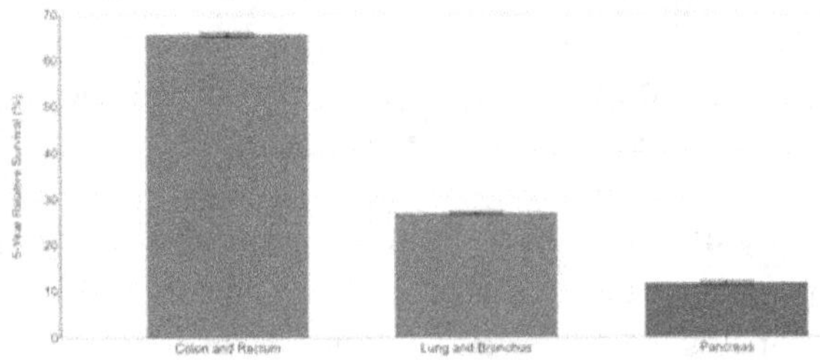

A recent research study "found that pancreatic cancer incidence increased among both sexes between 2000 and 2018. However, a greater relative increase was observed among women younger than 55 years, especially among those aged 15 to 34 years."[18]

Four graphs from the study are shown below, data for men use an orange triangle [▲] and data for women a green circle [●]:

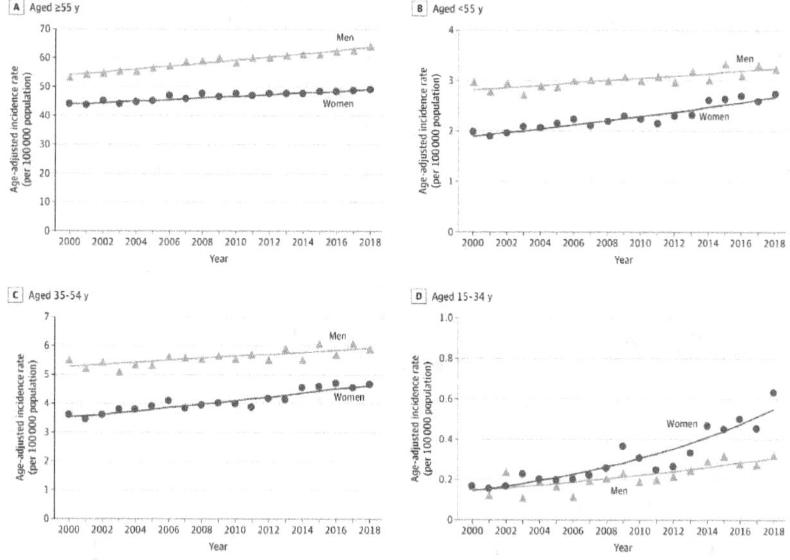

- The top left shows a relatively high incidence for men and women over 55 years old
- The top right shows a much lower but rising incidence for men and women under 55 years old
- The bottom left shows an increasing incidence for men and women aged 35 to 54 years old that is similar to men and women over 55 years
- The bottom right shows very low but rising incidence for 15 to 34 years old with a more rapidly rising curve for women relative to men.

The study authors acknowledge that "the reason for this relative increasing trend among younger women is unclear" and a "limitation of this study is the small number of patients with pancreatic cancer who were younger than 55 years" so further research is needed.

Finally, it's important to note that although advances in the early detection and treatment of pancreatic cancer have been slow-going, there have been an increasing number of therapies fielded since 2001. As stated in a 2021 presentation by Kim Reiss Binder, MD of the University of Pennsylvania:[19]

- There was no active therapy for pancreatic cancer up to 2001 and the survival rate was only 3 to 5 months.
- In 2001, Gemcitabine[20] was introduced and it took another decade until the drug Folfirinox[21] was launched in 2011
- From 2013 to 2020, an additional five therapies have been added, including three targeted therapies for specific patient types

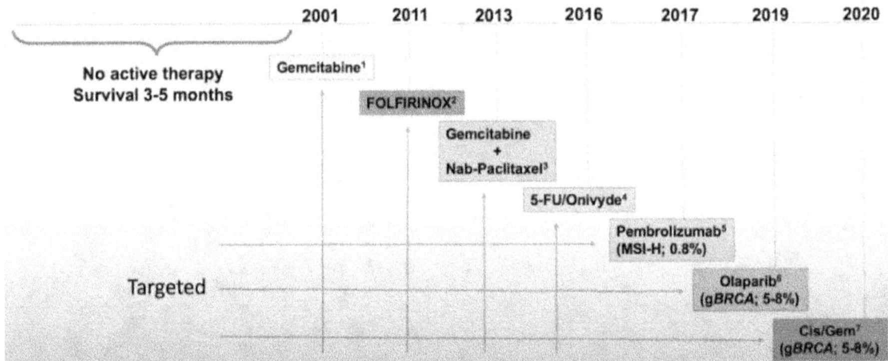

So, progress is being made that offers hope for more effective therapies for pancreatic cancer in the future. In the meantime, there are various treatment protocols available to patients, including the one I discuss in My Cancer Journey. Regarding new therapies in development, see The Long Road to New Drug Therapies and the link to the NIH Clinical Trials database in Suggested Resources, both of which are in the Appendices.

****

Okay, now you know a little more about cancer in general and that pancreatic cancer is a relatively rare but particularly nasty form of cancer. Let's move on to explanations of Procedures that you may encounter in your journey.

PROCEDURES

During the diagnostic and therapeutic monitoring of pancreatic cancer, you will likely encounter several common procedures such as ultrasound scan, CT scan, MRI scan, and endoscopy. Let's next take a look at the various procedures that are listed below, to which I'll be referring in the later section, My Cancer Journey.

Blood Workup

A blood workup involves taking a couple of tubes of blood that are then used to assess a variety of blood measures like white and red blood cell counts and indicators of liver and other organ performance. One particular measurement used to monitor pancreatic cancer is the cancer antigen 19-9 (CA19-9) blood test. According to the Mayo Clinic[22] (bold is mine):

- The CA19-9 "test measures the amount of a protein called CA 19-9 (cancer antigen 19-9) in the blood. **CA 19-9 is a type of tumor marker.** Tumor markers are substances made by cancer cells or by normal cells in response to cancer in the body."
- Healthy people can have small amounts of CA 19-9 in their blood. **High levels of CA 19-9 are often a sign of pancreatic cancer.** But sometimes, high levels can indicate other types of cancer or certain noncancerous disorders, including cirrhosis and gallstones.
- Because high levels of CA 19-9 can mean different things, **the test is not used by itself to screen for or diagnose cancer.** It can help monitor the progress of your cancer and the effectiveness of cancer treatment.
- A CA 19-9 blood test may be used to:
    o Monitor pancreatic cancer and cancer treatment. CA 19-9 levels often go up as cancer spreads and go down as tumors shrink.
    o See if cancer has returned after treatment.
    o The test is sometimes used with other tests to help confirm or rule out cancer.

- You may need a CA 19-9 blood test if you've been diagnosed with pancreatic cancer or other types of cancer related to high levels of CA 19-9. These cancers include bile duct cancer, colon cancer, and stomach cancer.
- Your health care provider may test you regularly to see if your cancer treatment is working. You may also be tested after your treatment is complete to see if the cancer has come back.

Ultrasound Scan

Ultrasound scans use sound to non-invasively look inside the body. According to Cancer Research UK:[23]

- Ultrasound scans use high-frequency sound waves to create a picture of a part of the body.
- An abdominal ultrasound scan shows up blood flow and changes in your tummy (abdomen), including abnormal growths.
- You might have this test to find out if you have pancreatic cancer or to see how big it is and whether it has spread.
- It can show changes or abnormal areas in your pancreas and liver.
- You are most likely to have this test if you have yellowing of the skin or eyes (jaundice) and your doctor needs to see if the bile ducts are blocked.
- The ultrasound scanner has a transducer that produces sound waves. The sound waves bounce off the organs inside your body, and the transducer also picks them up. The transducer links to a computer that turns the sound waves into a picture on the screen.
- Ultrasound scans are completely painless. You usually have the scan in the hospital x-ray department by a sonographer. A sonographer is a trained professional who is specialized in ultrasound scanning.
- An ultrasound scan is a very safe procedure. It doesn't involve radiation and there are usually no side effects.

CT Scan

CT scans use x-ray to non-invasively look inside the body with greater detail than ultrasound scans. According to Cancer Research UK[24],

- A computerized tomography (CT) scan combines a series of X-ray images taken from different angles around your body and uses computer processing to create cross-sectional images (slices) of the bones, blood vessels, and soft tissues inside your body. CT scan images provide more-detailed information than plain X-rays do.
- A CT scan has many uses, but it's particularly well-suited to quickly examine people who may have internal injuries from car accidents or other types of trauma. A CT scan can be used to visualize nearly all parts of the body and is used to diagnose disease or injury as well as to plan medical, surgical, or radiation treatment.
- Your doctor may recommend a CT scan to help:
  - Diagnose muscle and bone disorders, such as bone tumors and fractures
  - Pinpoint the location of a tumor, infection, or blood clot
  - Guide procedures such as surgery, biopsy, and radiation therapy
  - Detect and monitor diseases and conditions such as cancer, heart disease, lung nodules, and liver masses
  - Monitor the effectiveness of certain treatments, such as cancer treatment

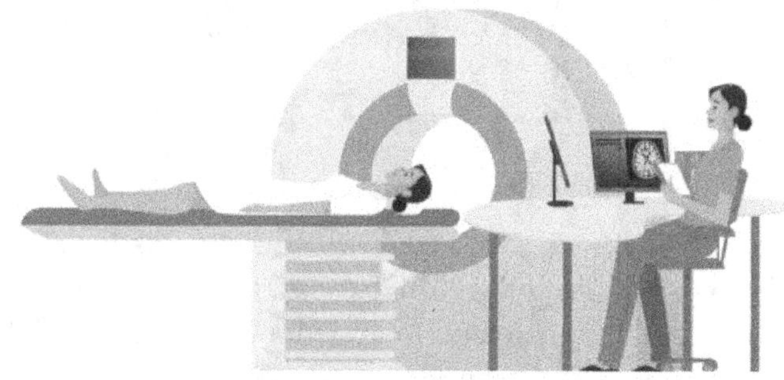

The figure above shows a typical CT scanner. The patient lies on a table that is then moved into the ring of the CT scanner that contains the x-ray generator. The scan is quick, even if contrast dye is used, and relatively quiet. The patient doesn't feel anything as the CT scanner collects and analyzes data.

MRI Scan

MRI scans use magnetic fields to non-invasively look inside the body with greater detail than CT scans. According to the Mayo Clinic,[25]

- Magnetic resonance imaging (MRI) is a medical imaging technique that uses a magnetic field and computer-generated radio waves to create detailed images of the organs and tissues in your body.
- Most MRI machines are large, tube-shaped magnets.
- When you lie inside an MRI machine, the magnetic field temporarily realigns water molecules in your body.
- Radio waves cause these aligned atoms to produce faint signals, which are used to create cross-sectional MRI images – like slices in a loaf of bread.
- The MRI machine can also produce 3D images that can be viewed from different angles.

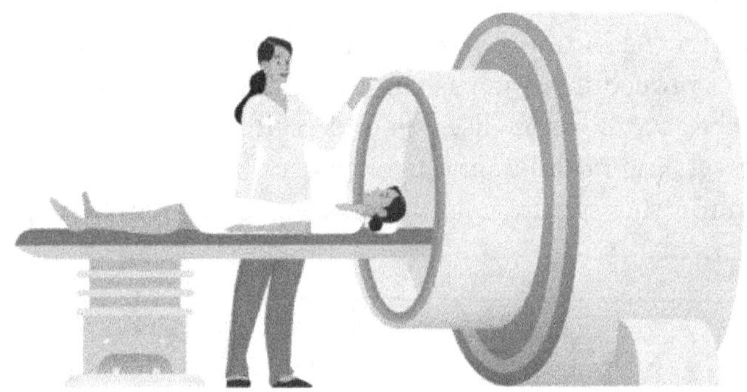

The figure above shows a typical MRI scanner. Like the CT scanner, the patient lies on a table that is then moved into the ring of the MRI scanner that contains the magnetic field generator. The ring is longer and narrower than the CT scanner ring. Some patients may feel claustrophobic when inside the ring, but a sedative may be requested if needed. Due to the noise the MRI machine generates during its use, the patient will be given ear plugs or a headset that reduces noise, enables the patient to hear the technician, and provides calming music that the patient selects.

The MRI scan takes longer than a CT scan, but the result is images that are more precise and clearer. The patient doesn't feel anything as the MRI scanner collects and analyzes data.

Upper Endoscopy

Endoscopy is a minimally invasive procedure that is performed with an instrument called an endoscope, "an illuminated usually fiber-optic flexible or rigid tubular instrument for visualizing the interior of a hollow organ or part (such as the bladder or esophagus) for diagnostic or therapeutic purposes that typically has one or more channels to enable passage of instruments (such as forceps or scissors)."[26]

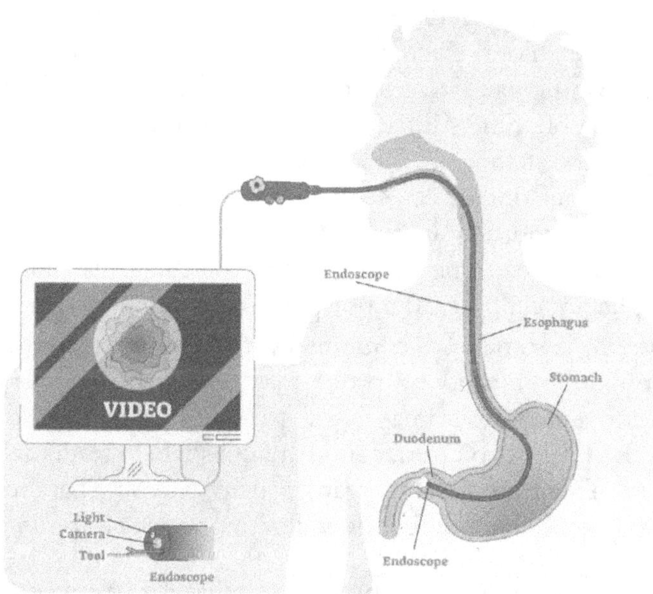

According to Mayo Clinic[27],

- An upper endoscopy is a procedure used to visually examine your upper digestive system with a tiny camera on the end of a long, flexible tube. A specialist in diseases of the digestive system

31

(gastroenterologist) uses endoscopy to diagnose and, sometimes, treat conditions that affect the esophagus, stomach, and beginning of the small intestine (duodenum).

- The medical term for an upper endoscopy is esophagogastroduodenoscopy. You may have an upper endoscopy done in your doctor's office, an outpatient surgery center, or a hospital.
- An upper endoscopy is used to diagnose and, sometimes, treat conditions that affect the upper part of your digestive system, including the esophagus, stomach, and beginning of the small intestine (duodenum).
- Your doctor may recommend an endoscopy procedure to:
  o Investigate symptoms. An endoscopy may help your doctor determine what's causing digestive signs and symptoms, such as nausea, vomiting, abdominal pain, difficulty swallowing, and gastrointestinal bleeding.
  o Diagnose. Your doctor may use endoscopy to collect tissue samples (biopsy) to test for diseases and conditions, such as anemia, bleeding, inflammation, diarrhea, or cancers of the digestive system.
  o Treat. Your doctor can pass special tools through the endoscope to treat problems in your digestive system, such as *cauterizing* (burning) a bleeding vessel to stop bleeding, widening a narrow esophagus, clipping off a polyp, or removing a foreign object.
- Endoscopy is sometimes combined with other procedures, such as an ultrasound. An ultrasound probe may be attached to the endoscope to create specialized images of the wall of your esophagus or stomach. Endoscopic ultrasound may also help your doctor create images of hard-to-reach organs, such as your pancreas. Newer endoscopes use high-definition video to provide clearer images.

There are two endoscopic procedures that I underwent which you may also encounter: EUS and ERCP.

Endoscopic Ultrasound (EUS)

EUS combines endoscopy with ultrasound. According to Mayo Clinic[28],

- Endoscopic ultrasound (EUS) is a minimally invasive procedure to assess digestive (gastrointestinal) and lung diseases.
- A special endoscope uses high-frequency sound waves to produce detailed images of the lining and walls of your digestive tract and chest, nearby organs such as the pancreas and liver, and lymph nodes.
- When combined with a procedure called fine-needle aspiration, EUS allows your doctor to sample (biopsy) fluid and tissue from your abdomen or chest for analysis.
- EUS with fine-needle aspiration can be a minimally invasive alternative to exploratory surgery.

Endoscopic Retrograde Cholangiopancreatography (ERCP)

ERCP is a minimally invasive procedure that combines endoscopy with x-ray. According to the National Institute of Diabetes and Digestive and Kidney Diseases (NIDDK)[29],

- Endoscopic retrograde cholangiopancreatography (ERCP) is a procedure that combines upper gastrointestinal (GI) endoscopy and x-rays to treat problems of the bile and pancreatic ducts.
- During ERCP, the doctor
  - locates the opening where the bile and pancreatic ducts empty into the duodenum
  - slides a thin, flexible tube called a catheter through the endoscope and into the ducts
  - injects a special dye, also called contrast medium, into the ducts through the catheter to make the ducts more visible on x-rays
  - uses a type of x-ray imaging, called fluoroscopy, to examine the ducts and look for narrowed areas or blockages
- The doctor may pass tiny tools through the endoscope to
  - open blocked or narrowed ducts
  - break up or remove stones
  - perform a biopsy or remove tumors in the ducts
  - insert stents – tiny tubes that a doctor leaves in narrowed ducts to hold them open

Infusion Access Port

To facilitate the administration of repeated chemotherapy, an infusion access port is used. The access port provides a convenient way to administer drugs rather than to make multiple punctures in the veins of a patient's arms or back of the hands. As shown below, the access port consists of a little cup with a durable top that can take repeated needle sticks over months or years. Leading out of this cup is a thin tube that carries the infused drug to the patient.

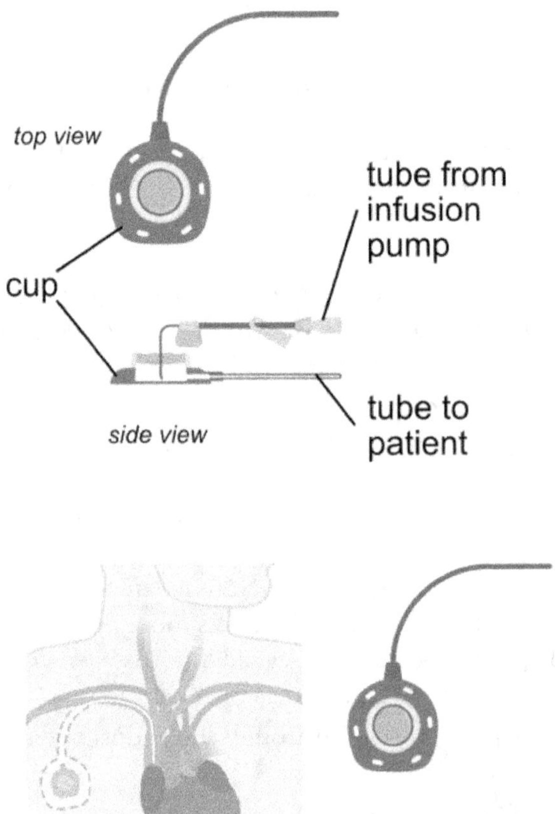

The cup is inserted under the skin of the chest and the tube is threaded under the skin, over the collar bone, and into a vein that leads to the heart (shown above). Once installed, the port may be accessed by inserting a special port mating needle, through the chest skin and into the access port cup (shown lower right). These ports are available as *power*

ports that can accept large flows such as contrast dye that is used during certain CT and MRI scans. The insertion of the mating needle through the chest skin does cause a prick, but creams are available that will reduce the discomfort.

External Infusion Pump

Infusion access ports are primarily used to deliver medication from an external infusion pump, although they may also be used to deliver fluids, contrast dyes, and obtain blood samples. According to the Food and Drug Administration (FDA)[30],

- An external infusion pump is a medical device used to deliver fluids into a patient's body in a controlled manner. There are many different types of infusion pumps, which are used for a variety of purposes and in a variety of environments.
- Infusion pumps may be capable of delivering fluids in large or small amounts and may be used to deliver nutrients or medications – such as insulin or other hormones, antibiotics, chemotherapy drugs, and pain relievers.
- Hospital infusion pumps are designed for use at a patient's bedside. Others, called ambulatory infusion pumps, are designed to be portable or wearable so drugs can be delivered as the patient moves about outside of the hospital.

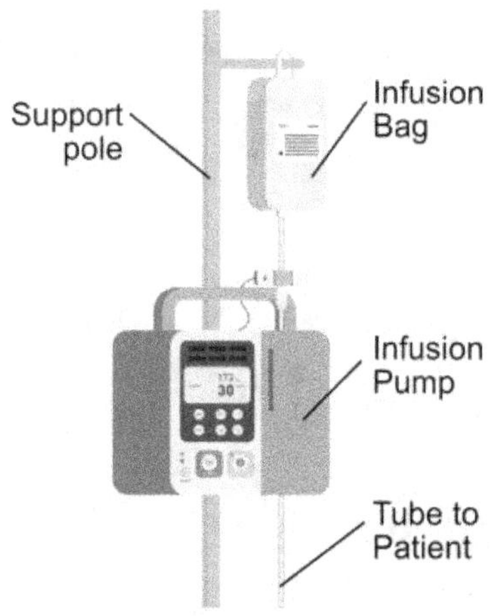

The illustration above shows the parts of a typical hospital infusion pump setup.

- A support pole is used to attach the required items for infusion; this pole has a wheeled base so the entire setup can be easily moved about.
- The infusion bag is hung on a support pole hook and holds the infusion drugs that are delivered to the patient.
- The tubing from the infusion bag passes through the infusion pump which is programmed to deliver the drug at the correct rate and for the right amount of time.
- The tube exits the infusion pump and is connected to the patient's access port.

Portable infusion pumps contain both the infusion bag and a small infusion pump that fits inside a bag with a shoulder strap similar to a fanny pack. This design enables drugs to be infused at the patient's home. I discuss the portable infusion pump further ahead under the section, Two-Week Therapy Cycle, Home Infusion.

***

Now that you have a general understanding of procedures that you may encounter, let's move on to my own cancer journey story where I share some more facts, personal insights, and thoughts with you.

MY CANCER JOURNEY (SO FAR)

Now that I've provided the general background on cancer and procedures, I'll continue with a timeline of how my cancer was diagnosed and the start of my therapy.

> Note that while there is certainly common ground among all cancer patients, every cancer patient's journey is different. Your kind of cancer, how your cancer was detected, the stage of your cancer when detected, the therapies that you receive, and your tolerance and response to therapy – all define your journey. There is no one-size-fits-all story, and my story is intended solely to offer my own experience and insights that may be helpful to the reader.

The diagram below shows where I was in my journey when I completed this book – just entering the 7th of 12 two-week therapy cycles. Barring the unforeseen, I will complete my current therapy in October – just in time to celebrate Diane's birthday and our wedding anniversary (both occurring on Halloween).

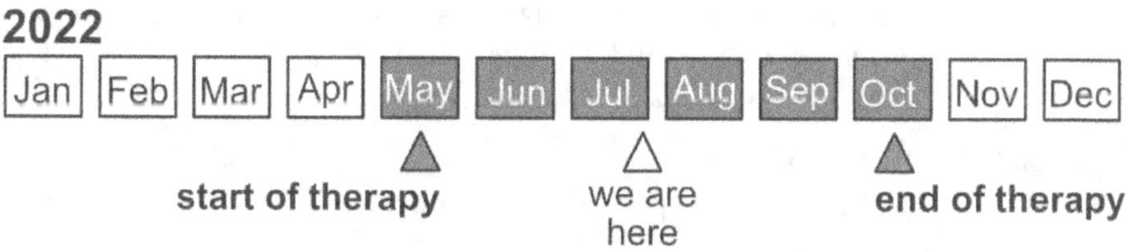

The table below briefly outlines those key events in my journey up to this point in chronological order. The table is followed by my narrative which gives more details.

Key Events

Date	Event
01/13/22	Annual wellness check; normal (as usual)
02/18/22	Presented to primary care physician (PCP) with a complaint of abdominal pain
03/15/22	Symptoms were not better, PCP referred me to a gastroenterologist (GI) specialist
03/28/22	CT scan ordered in preparation for the GI specialist visit
04/11/22	CT reveals with 3 cm mass within the head of the pancreas most in keeping with a primary pancreatic neoplasm (*tumor*). Recommendation to assess with contrast-enhanced magnetic resonance imaging (MRI) or endoscopic ultrasound (EUS).
04/18/22	CT CAP (pancreatic protocol) with pancreatic head mass suspicious for pancreatic adenocarcinoma; multiple sub-centimeter hepatic lesions not seen on outside CT which are indeterminate but suspicious for metastasis; vascular involvement with short segment distortion of the portal vein/SMV
04/18/22	Seen at Duke clinic by my medical and surgical oncologists. Recommended MRI to further characterize liver lesions, and FOLFIRINOX therapy pending MRI
04/18/22	CA19-9 value of 6,908 vs. a normal range of 0-37 units per milliliter.
04/18/22	Magnetic resonance imaging (MRI) reveals the liver with multiple small hepatic metastases (*cancer that has spread from the pancreas to the liver*); indeterminate osseous (*boney*) lesion in the T9 vertebral body (*middle of the spine*); pancreatic head mass
04/20/22	Biopsy via endoscopic ultrasound (EUS) and fine needle aspiration (FNA) positive for adenocarcinoma
04/26/22	Infusion port placed
04/27/22	The first dose of FOLFIRINOX - full doses of all agents
05/02/22	Presented to the emergency department (ED) after syncopal episode (*fainting*) and given fluids (see Dehydration in the *Bumps in the Road* section)

Date	Event
05/12/22	Dose #2 FOLFIRINOX was delayed due to Absolute Neutrophil Count (ANC), a blood test that checks for red and white cells and platelets
5/23/22 – 5/25/22	Hospitalized for elevated liver enzymes; stricture in one of my biliary ducts. Placement of endoscopic stent into the biliary/pancreatic duct (see Bile Duct Obstruction in the *Bumps in the Road* section)
5/28/22	Return to ED with severe chest pain (see Chest Pain in the *Bumps in the Road* section
7/26/22	Pancreas: a dedicated mass measures 1.5 x 1.7 cm previously 2.7 x 2.6 cm (2; 141). There is an adjacent moderately severe narrowing of the SMV, with adjacent collaterals[31]. Liver: Similar small poorly defined hepatic lesions are better appreciated on previous MRI. No new lesions. The portal and hepatic veins are patent (not obstructed).
7/28/22	Start my 7th of 12 two-week rounds of chemotherapy. Morning blood work revealed that my CA19-9 was down from 10,120 a month ago to 1,912 (normal is 0-37). Spoke with our physician to discuss my CT and CA19-9. Although the results are positive, it is not possible to know with confidence how the chemotherapy will perform over the next 3-months (the completion of my therapy).

Note that I constructed the table above by using the entries in my patient portal. In retrospect, it would have been helpful for me to keep a daily journal. Fortunately, in addition to Diane's reliable memory, she also maintains a log of events and questions/answers with my health care team. A simple, hand-written daily journal example is provided below.

Date/Time	Event	Action Taken
7/15/2022 8:30 am	Upset stomach after breakfast	Alka-Seltzer taken and seemed to relieve the discomfort
7/16/2022 noon	A good appetite for lunch	Had a hardy soup with tuna sandwich after taking Creon and no problems
7/18/2022 8:30 am	Experienced burning pain in my hands when taking a bag of frozen vegatables	Sent a message to my healthcare team via my patient portal and was recommended to use oven mitts. They will discuss mitigation further at my next visit

First Signs of Trouble

As you can see from the key events table above, my journey started in February of 2022 when I began to experience abdominal pain after eating that would radiate into my chest and around to my back. I've had back spasms in the past that were severe enough to collapse me into unconsciousness. This new pain, however, was something else – deep and persistent, so I set up an appointment with my primary care physician (PCP).

After his examination, my PCP felt that my problem was a fairly common gastrointestinal issue due to inadequate fiber and water consumption. I assured him that while I was definitely not drinking the recommended 64 ounces of water daily, I was eating high-fiber foods daily and staying away from high-fat, high-calorie choices.

My PCP recommended that I use over-the-counter fiber supplements and drink plenty of water – that if I pushed ahead, the problem would resolve itself and if not, then we could look for other plausible causes of my discomfort. I followed his advice, but the symptoms only worsened into March to the point where it was significantly affecting my quality of life and my work performance.

I informed my physician that things were getting worse and asked that he request a consult with a gastroenterologist (GI) specialist. I took the earliest appointment which was a couple of months into the future. I then asked if there was some kind of diagnostic test that could be performed before the visit with the GI specialist that would help in the diagnosis and my PCP ordered a CT scan – the earliest appointment was a month into the future.

The pain I was experiencing had increased to the point where it was affecting my focus and the quality of my work. I learned that I could reduce the pain by eating more small meals rather than the conventional three daily meals. Having some small control over my discomfort helped me to refocus and have less painful days.

Diagnosis

Initial Assessment

My CT scan was performed in April, and my PCP called to tell me that he had "bad news," specifically, that a tumor of about three centimeters (about 1 $^{3/16}$ inch) was located on the head of my pancreas. This smallish tumor represented about 40% of the approximately 6-inch-long pancreas.

> An initial misdiagnosis of pancreatic cancer is typical because the symptoms are so similar to GI problems. Physicians reasonably look for the most common origin first and then other less commonplace reasons. If, for example, you are having a headache, then your physician would likely advise a non-prescriptive drug like aspirin, Aleve®, or Advil® first and not rush to have your brain scanned in search of a tumor.

There aren't any current methods to adequately screen for pancreatic cancer. The CA19-9 measurement to which I referred above is used during the treatment of pancreatic cancer as a trending indicator; however, this test has been deemed unreliable as a screening tool. Some physicians view the Prostate Specific Antigen (PSA) test in a similar light.[32]

Short of finding a pancreatic tumor by happenstance – as was the case with Supreme Court Justice Ruth Bader Ginsburg[33], pancreatic cancer can grow silently and undetected for years. Consequently, by the time someone experiences the abdominal and back pain I described, jaundice, and other signs the disease has already established a beachhead and is making its way into other organs.

With my revised diagnosis, Diane immediately initiated her nurse-advocate role on my behalf. She spoke directly with my PCP to inform him that my care forward-going would be managed at Duke. She told my PCP whom to call at Duke, and also made her own calls within Duke to ensure a smooth transition of my medical information and care plan.

Within days I was meeting with a surgical oncologist (who would advise us on surgical removal of the tumor), a medical oncologist (who would advise us on chemotherapy), and various other health care team members like physician assistants and nurses.

A major concern that Diane and my health care team had was my unintentional loss of weight. Between my annual wellness check in January and these first meetings with my health care team in April, my weight dropped from 159 pounds to 149 pounds (by June my weight would drop to 138 pounds and later to 133 pounds). The view of my health care team, however, was very encouraging.

We never had a discussion with my physicians about the stage of my disease. Rather, my health care team's focus was on treating the disease in its current state with an aggressive "gold standard" program and making modifications depending on how I was managing the therapy and how the disease responded to the therapy.

I felt then and today that working with this tightly knit and determined team of medical experts would give me the best chance to fight my disease.

Follow-up Assessments & Procedures

My Duke health care team scheduled follow-up assessments of my initial CT to confirm the diagnosis including:

- A Blood Workup was conducted, including the CA19-9.

- Another CT scan confirmed the location and size of the tumor, and also indicated three or four spots in my liver.

- An MRI scan provided more detail of my pancreas and liver in three dimensions, clearly showing that the pancreatic tumor was encasing my superior mesenteric vein (SMV). The SMV is a large blood vessel in the abdomen that drains blood from the small intestine, the first sections of the large intestine, and other digestive organs.

Armed with the non-invasive information from my CA19-9, CT, and MRI, my health care team scheduled an Endoscopic Ultrasound (EUS) as described under the Procedures section above. During this procedure, biopsy samples of both the tumor and one of the spots in my liver (*metastasis* or *mets*) were obtained. These samples provided the final confirmation that the tumor and a sample met in my liver was malignant. Although my surgical oncologist felt he could address the SMV encasement, the liver mets ruled out a surgical solution for me.

Steven Merlin notes that "CT scans are the preferred method when examining the lungs as they provide much better imaging and resolution in lung tissue over an MRI scan. Sometimes patients prefer having an MRI over a CT scan and will get pushback from a radiologist if they request an MRI for examining the chest."

My Departure Plan and Housecleaning

The day that my diagnosis was confirmed I sat down at my computer and drafted my *departure plan* – a list of action items I would need to take in light of my diagnosis. Taking time to write a departure plan might seem like an odd thing to do but I realized that things could go very badly very quickly. I wanted to ensure that I removed a variety of obstacles that Diane would face in my absence. My plan not only reflected my need to take reasonable action but was personally empowering (more on this in the Philosophical Perspectives section). I wrote the plan as a simple, bulleted list and in roughly chronological order that included:

☐ Speak with our financial planner so he knew that our short- and long-term assumptions had changed

☐ Update an Excel Projection that I had created to augment the work of our financial planner
☐ Turn off auto-renew for my consulting WordPress website and business Gmail account
☐ Clean up my personal and business Gmail files
☐ Copy and organize key information onto a thumb drive so it was convenient for Diane (e.g., wills and advance health care directives)
☐ Clean up and organize my Microsoft and Google cloud drives
☐ Change the account information for our Microsoft Live and Office accounts
☐ Provide Diane with my passwords vault so she will be able to access my various online accounts and secure notes
☐ Change information for autopay and deposit links (e.g., checking account, Venmo account)
☐ Create a family, friends, and associates email list so Diane could send out notices
☐ Cancel auto-renewal for services like Zoom and my online calendar scheduling app
☐ Explore hospice care (external vs. home) under Medicare A
☐ Conclude funeral arrangements
☐ Collect my insurance policy
☐ Distribute certain personal effects to select individuals that were not stipulated in my will (e.g., books, camera gear) and dispose of other personal effects via sale or donation (e.g., musical instrument)
☐ Stop various payments: Medicare, auto insurance, and credit cards
☐ Keep my cell phone active for a year after my departure to ensure that Diane would receive any dual authentication requests.

I also generated a written brief of the financial plan that Diane and I had created and were following, including details on what my personal projection model was forecasting over the next ten to twenty years. I hoped that this information would be a handy reminder to Diane that by sticking to our retirement plan she would help ensure that she had the necessary resources throughout her life.

I also updated my LinkedIn profile to "retired," started shutting down my consulting website and aggressively unsubscribed from the various email newsletters that I followed. One of the effects of this activity was that my daily email load was greatly reduced. I found myself checking email and feeling a little isolated by a nearly empty inbox. However, my need to be constantly connected was no longer pressing for me and I came to enjoy the near absence of insistent message notice *pings* on my phone.

I next created a shopping list on Amazon of articles that I thought I might need during therapy. One assumption I made was that my health would rapidly degrade during therapy to the point where I would need a lot of assistance. Some of the items I placed on the list were skull caps (assuming I would quickly go bald), travel vomit bags (assuming I would encounter a lot of nausea), and an intercom system (assuming I might need assistance in the middle of the night and would have to alert Diane who sleeps in a different room – see Toxicity of Chemotherapy in the Appendices). At the halfway point in my therapy, I haven't needed any of these expected items.

Finally, I set about housecleaning to clear away the junk that had slowly accumulated over the years. This involved going through numerous storage boxes and tossing out items that no longer had use or meaning. Included in the purge was a stack of books I had used for journaling over the years. These journals were a kind of therapy, writing down what was in my mind so I could better see unfounded assumptions and biased judgment at the time. I never looked back to the journals, and honestly would have trouble reading my handwriting or remembering the context at the time I made the entries.

The housecleaning exercise also uncovered many nice memories, including old photographs of family and friends, and annual Father's Day cards that our daughter gave me over the years. Her cards were funny, irreverent, and always appreciated. I put those cards back into safe storage.

Therapy

With a surgical option off of the table, my medical oncologist determined that the appropriate therapy for me was chemotherapy without radiation. The hope was that the chemotherapy would reduce the size of my pancreatic tumor and liver mets, possibly improve my quality of life, and (perhaps) open the door to a surgical procedure at a future date. Following are some key features of the chemotherapy that I'm receiving.

Chemotherapy Prep and Cycle

My program runs in two-week intervals over twelve weeks for a total of six months that will conclude around October 2022, barring the unforeseen. The protocol incorporates three different chemotherapy drugs: Oxaliplatin, Irinotecan, and Fluorouracil (5FU) (see Drug Reference in Appendices).

Infusion Access Port

To facilitate the administration of repeated chemotherapy infusions, an infusion port was surgically implanted on the right side of my chest a couple of inches below my collar bone. The port provides a convenient way to obtain blood samples and administer drugs rather than to make multiple punctures in my hands and arms.

The details for an infusion access port are provided in Infusion Access Port under the Procedures section. The type of port that I received is commonly called a "power port" and can accept large flows such as hydration fluids and contrast dye used for CT and MRI scans.

The placement of my infusion access port was performed under light anesthesia. I was awake during the procedure but felt nothing – not the scalpel that cut open a pocket in my chest for the port, or the threading of the tube from the port over my collar bone and into a vein that led into my heart. The incision on my chest was closed with medical glue that wore off over time. The day after the procedure the surgical site was slightly sore, but that sensation passed by the following day.

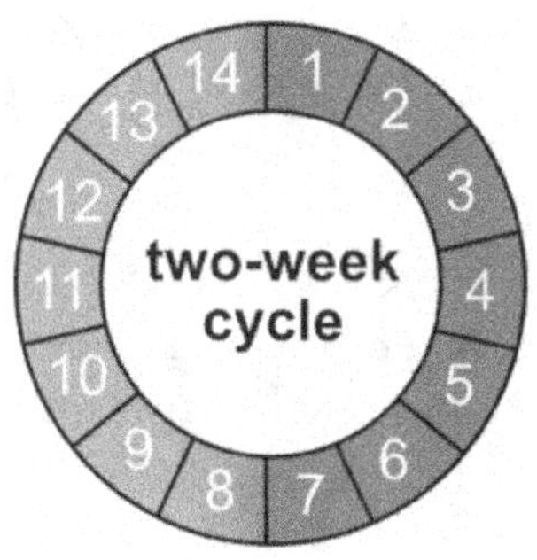

Day 1

Each two-week cycle begins with a visit to the hospital where I have blood drawn. The results of the blood draw inform my health care team if there may be any reason to postpone the therapy session. A postponement of one week did occur on one occasion when a low white blood cell count was detected. The delay enabled me to receive a drug to help generate white blood cells (*Pegfilgrastim-bmez*) and for the drug to take effect.

Occasionally, a CA19-9 (described under Blood Workup above) is ordered to assess if there is a change in the cancer activity. The normal CA 19-9 range in a healthy person is 0-37 units per milliliter. My initial CA19-9 reading was 6,900. Subsequent CA19-9 tests conducted during my therapy peaked at 10,000 and then dropped to 1,920 at the halfway point of my therapy. Ideally, the CA19-9 results will continue to trend down in the weeks ahead.

Also, throughout my therapy, additional CT scans will be occasionally performed to take a closer look at changes in the tumor size and for evidence of further metastases.

The Solo Journeyers

A few thoughts about those who may be making their cancer journey with little or no support. I noticed these individuals during my very first visits to Duke Hospital and I see them on my return visits.

People from all levels of society who are obviously infirmed, standing in a check-in line alone. People waiting their turn slumped in a chair, staring into space, or with their heads bowed as if in prayer. The elderly wife slowly pushes her elderly husband in a wheelchair, a silent testimonial to their marriage vows. I wonder how these people manage their journeys.

How far do they travel? How do they make their way to the hospital and back home again? How do they pilot the many hospital nooks and crannies to make their appointments on time? How do they navigate the insurance issues? With whom do they share their hopes and fears?

I am reminded of how remarkably fortunate I am to have the support of family and friends, and I don't know how I would manage my journey alone. I hope that the reader has the support that she needs and deserves, and I look to the day when insurance covers the cost of nurse advocates for patients with life-threatening diseases like cancer.

In the meantime, if you or someone you know needs transportation to cancer therapy, then see the American Cancer Society *Road to Recovery* program at
https://www.cancer.org/support-programs-and-services/road-to-recovery.html

Hospital Infusion

The first two chemotherapy drugs are infused into me under nurse supervision at the hospital. The setting for these infusions is a nice room with a comfortable therapy chair, a television, and a separate chair for a designated visitor during the treatment.

I'm always accompanied by Diane who provides companionship and assistance as needed. Diane can work on her Duke projects via her laptop as my infusions are delivered. The picture below is from one of my Day 1 infusions at the hospital, note the infusion pump on the wheeled stand between my chair and the guest chair. As you can see, the treatment environment is laid back with a window for natural lighting and a view of the outside. Also, note the blanket that is heated – a welcome amenity when your weight is well below normal, and you are more likely to feel cold.

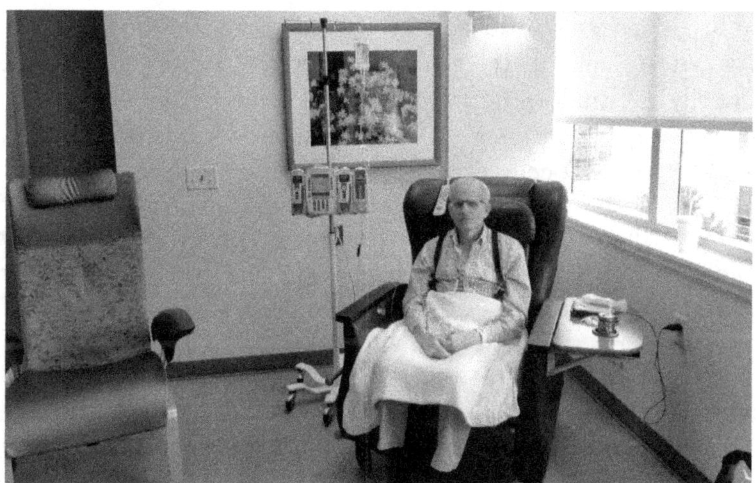

Before infusing any chemotherapy, the attending nurse will administer an antinausea drug. Occasionally, I will also receive fluids to help me maintain hydration.

When handling the chemotherapy drugs, the nurse follows a strict garment protocol that included a disposable coat and two layers of gloves. These precautions are taken due to the toxic nature of the chemotherapy from which health care workers must be isolated. See

<u>Toxicity of Chemotherapy</u> under the Drug Reference section in the Appendices for more information.

The first drug infusion of Oxaliplatin takes about two hours, and the second drug infusion of Irinotecan takes about ninety minutes. Typically, it's a five-hour day at the hospital, including setup, change of drugs, adjustment of the infusion pump, transfer to the portable infusion pump, and cleanup. Add the commute time between Duke Hospital and our home and it's a long day indeed, however, some other cancer patients travel much further to be treated at Duke.

Some of the side effects that I've experienced on these drugs include pain in my jaw muscles when eating certain foods or drinking certain beverages. I can also have difficulties articulating my words, and my voice becomes hoarse and softer – so communicating with people, even those nearby can be a challenge. These effects wear off over a few hours.

The drugs have also caused *trigger finger* where one finger may decide on its own to fully extend itself while the others remain at rest. Occasionally my middle finger straightens, and I believe it is my body sending a *salute* to my cancer. These effects are likely from the first drug infused and typically occur as the second infusion drug is started.

Before starting the Irinotecan infusion, I'm given atropine to prevent abdominal cramps. Fortunately, my health care providers have helped manage nausea and diarrhea neither of which I have yet experienced as a consequence of my therapy.

Before departing the hospital, a nurse disconnects the hospital infusion pump and connects a portable infusion pump that accompanies me home. This portable pump is connected to a bag of Fluorouracil (5FU) and the pump is programmed to deliver the drug over 46 hours. The pump and drug bag are contained in a small carry bag that is suspended from my shoulder.

At the end of the hospital infusion, I'm typically fatigued and need to have Diane push me on a wheelchair to our car for the ride home. The majority of the fatigue is caused by the medications and part is likely the effects of a long day.

As I approached the halfway mark of my treatments, I started to experience the cumulative effects of the chemotherapy, specifically, neuropathy (numbness in my fingers and toes), and sensitivity in my mouth and lips. For the sixth round of chemotherapy, my hospital infusions were reduced by about 20%. Curiously, my *recovery* after the portable pump was removed was slower than in the past and I experienced a loss of taste that made eating another task to survive rather than a pleasurable event.

Home Infusion

Days 2-3

The portable infusion pump runs for about two days to deliver the Fluorouracil (5FU). I know it's working properly via a green, flashing indicator light and also an occasional *whooshing* noise it makes as the pump delivers the medication. It took some initial trial-and-error for me to figure out how to move about and sleep with the pump bag over my shoulder. After the first couple of chemotherapy rounds, however, it really hasn't presented any significant problem. Shown left in the image below is the portable infusion pump in the carry bag. During use, the carry bag also holds a small plastic bag of chemotherapy. Shown right is the portable pump ready to wear (pen included for dimensional reference).

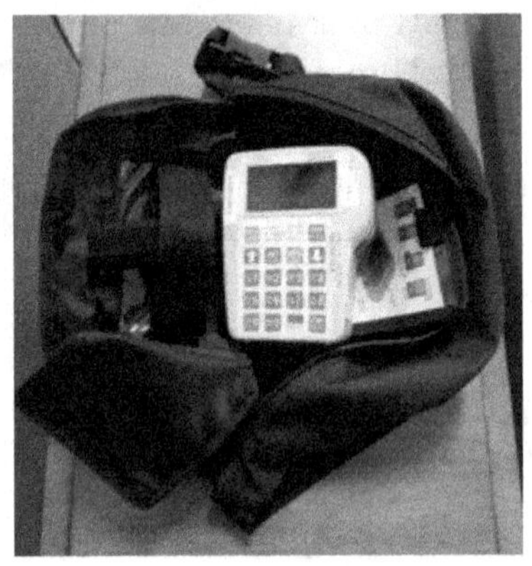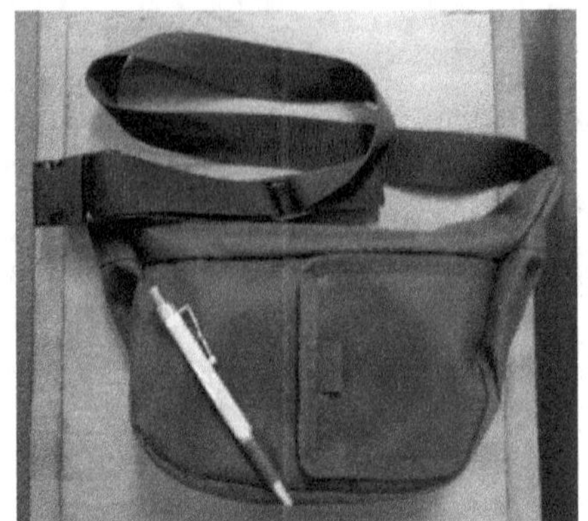

The access port connection to the pump is secured with a bandage and tape on my chest. I have the tube that runs from the pump into my access port under my tee shirt, and I to ensure that I'm not inadvertently getting the tube snagged on anything like my belt or knobs on kitchen drawers. The securing tape helps ensure that disconnection doesn't occur.

During the two days of home infusion, I regularly check to ensure that a leak hasn't occurred somewhere between the infusion bag and the access port. A leak is a serious problem in that it requires immediate action to limit the amount of drug lost which then creates a hazardous exposure to my family. Part of the home infusion kit that we receive includes hazmat items like a protective gown, gloves, and pads to absorb leaks. Thankfully, we haven't had a leak problem so far.

During the days of home infusion and for a couple of days after the infusion is completed, I refrain from direct contact with my family to help ensure that I'm not exposing them to the chemotherapy that my body is voiding (see Toxicity of Chemotherapy in the Appendices). I must even avoid handling our canine companion who seems to know that something's not right, including the fact that I'm keeping my distance.

After the home infusion is finished, Diane completes a "take down" of the infusion pump. This process includes shutting the pump off, disconnecting the line from the pump to my infusion port, drawing blood from the infusion port to ensure blood flow, flushing the infusion port with saline, flushing the infusion port with heparin (a drug that keeps blood from clotting the infusion port), and removing the needle from the infusion pump line into my infusion port. All of the items used to connect me to the chemotherapy are placed into a special, bright yellow and clearly marked plastic hazmat container that safely isolates the therapy items from our home. Diane applies a waterproof bandage over my infusion port so I can shower without exposing the needle site – I remove the bandage in a day or two.

My level of fatigue, energy, and appetite tend to fluctuate during the at-home infusion due in part to a steroid (Dexamethasone) that I receive. The steroid is an anti-inflammatory against Irinotecan administration and boosts energy for a few days after which fatigue sets in. Consequently, I have periods when I feel more normal and energetic followed by periods when I need to sleep.

Days 3-6

Post Hospital Injection

Because I had experienced a reduction in my white blood cell count early in my therapy, I was prescribed a follow-up injection. A couple of days after completing the home infusion I return to the hospital to receive Pegfilgrastim-bmez, a growth factor used to prevent low white blood cell count (*neutropenia*). This injection is administered on the underside of my upper arm. Although one of the common side effects is bone pain, I haven't experienced any problems so far.

Days 7-14

Once I'm past the mid-point of a two-week cycle, I generally start to feel more normal. During days 7-14 my focus and energy tend to improve, and I can perform more physical and mental tasks. Note that as I entered the halfway point of my therapy, the recovery time from my infusions took longer than usual. Of course, all good things end, and on Day 14, I prepare myself to return to the hospital the following morning and start another two-week therapy cycle with all of its challenges and side effects.

The Day to Day

My daily activities that start on Day 1 of my therapy cycle continue throughout the full fourteen days of the cycle. I make my best efforts to eat enough calories to maintain my weight, have a little exercise if just pacing and simple strength training, and enjoy the little pleasures in life.

During Days 1-5 my morning starts off with a regimen of various pills to help reduce acid indigestion (24-hour Nexium), help ensure that I get the nutrition from what I eat (Creon), a steroid to quiet my stomach, and provide a little energy, an anti-nausea drug, Miralax to help keep my GI system in line, and a potassium supplement. The image below is an example of a typical morning dosing.

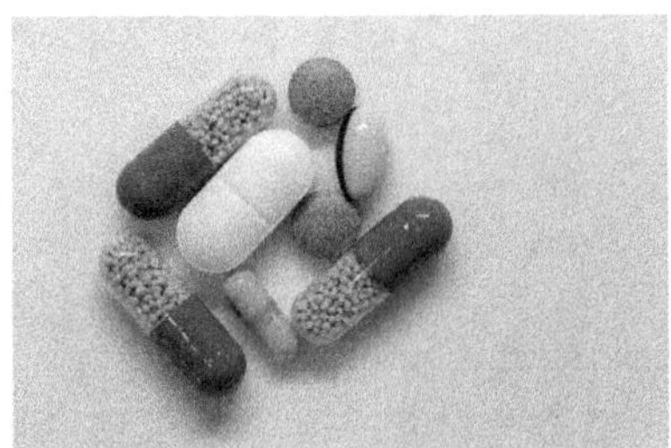

On researching Creon for this book, I encountered some differences in opinion about when, exactly, to take my Creon prescription. The directions for use state only that Creon should be taken during a meal. Should the full dose be taken before the first bite? Should the Creon dose be ingested during the meal, so it becomes sandwiched in with the food to release enzymes more evenly?

I've been taking the full 3-capsule dose before my first bite of food which seems (anecdotally) to work for me. I also tried spreading out the full dose throughout a meal. For example, one capsule before my first bite, another capsule when I finish 1/3rd of my meal, and another capsule when I finish 2/3rd of my meal. This method seemed to achieve similar results.

Creon is a popular enzyme with no generic form that is expensive (see
What is the Doughnut Hole under the Appendices). Generally, after Day
5 I stop taking the steroid and anti-nausea meds.

During Days 3-6, the chemotherapy is more or less depleted from my
system via urine, stool, and sweat. In general, with every day that passes, I
feel more normal, gain interest in eating, and experience less fatigue. No
two cycles of therapy are identical, however, and my *recovery* time from
the effects of chemotherapy can be a bit shorter or longer in each
following 2-week cycle.

The picture below shows a simple plastic container we use to keep my
various drugs organized and handy. Because chemo brain can create
confusion, I also advise you to keep a pad and pencil with the drugs. List
the drugs you will take on a given day, and cross off those drugs by
marking the time at which you took them. Using the pad not only
confirms for you that you haven't missed a drug or taken it twice, but if
you have a caretaker in your home like a spouse, then they are also in the
loop.

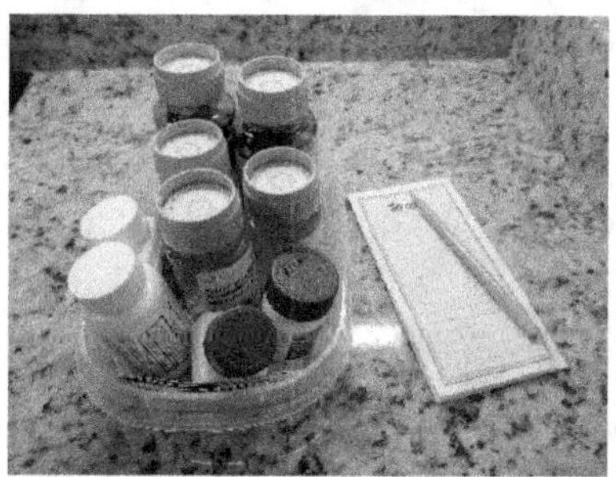

wouldn't know that he had any medical problems to look at him because he presented as a tough-as-nails kind of guy.

My mother kept track of my father's recommended diets and his growing home drug formulary, organizing his medications in a simple container like the one shown above. She would also take a list of my father's medications when he had a physician's appointment, surprising physicians with the variety and number of drugs that my father was consuming daily. Considering that my mother had no medical training, it's remarkable how good a job she did as my father's advocate.

Before my diagnosis, I was in good health and had no medical issues that required regular medication – no blood pressure meds, statins, insulin, etc. Now I think about my father's drug box and truly understand the situation that he and my mother endured for years.

Common Side Effects

I alluded to the side effects of chemotherapy above and now want to briefly comment on some of the more common ones that may concern you. For this section I've included excerpts of side effects provided on the Canadian Cancer Society (CCS) website[35] in quotes, followed by my personal experience with these side effects. I also added some side effects that I did experience which were not included in the CCS source for common side effects. The CCS notes that,

> "Side effects can happen with any type of treatment, but not everyone has them or experiences them in the same way. If you develop side effects, they can happen any time during, immediately after or a few days or weeks after chemotherapy. Sometimes late side effects develop months or years after chemotherapy. Most side effects go away on their own or can be treated, but some side effects may last a long time or become permanent."

Fatigue

"Fatigue makes a person feel more tired than usual and can interfere with daily activities and sleep. Fatigue may be caused by anemia, specific chemotherapy drugs, poor appetite, or depression. It may also be related to toxic substances that are made in the body when cancer cells break down and die. Fatigue can happen within days after a chemotherapy treatment and can last long after treatment ends. It also tends to be worse when you are having other treatments, such as radiation therapy. Fatigue usually gets better over time."

Fatigue has been the main side effect I've experienced. The severity of my fatigue has sometimes put me in a withdrawn state where I just needed to lie down and not engage with anyone. At other times, my fatigue has limited the amount of activity such as walking and reading. While I don't advocate forcing yourself to do anything when you are seriously fatigued, I have found that putting in a little effort can help improve energy levels. For example, on those days when I don't want to move but make a little effort to do so, I generally feel better both physically and emotionally.

Changes in Taste and Smell

"Some chemotherapy drugs can affect taste buds causing changes in taste. For example, you may find that meats have a metallic taste. Even foods that you normally crave, such as sweet or salty snacks, can taste bad. You may become more sensitive to smells. Smells that others don't notice may make you nauseous. It can take months for both the sense of smell and taste to return to normal after chemotherapy."

I've experienced both taste and scent side effects. It is remarkable to me that even plain water can have an *off* taste at times. Although my sense of smell is not that great to begin with, there are times when I seem to have a heightened sensitivity to scents. Occasionally, I feel as though I can smell the chemotherapy on my skin – seeing the reaction of Ozzie, our canine companion, to me during therapy, he certainly seems to be able to detect an unusual scent. I've also noticed how some hand soaps seem to have a stronger than usual scent.

My recommendation on the scent issue is to try to replace any product that has a scent with substitutes that have no scent profile (e.g., hand soaps, laundry detergent). At the same time, you may want to experiment with scents that you find appealing while experiencing scent side effects (e.g., fresh flowers, air fresheners). Some patients report that aroma therapy using essential oils helps (e.g., lavender, citrus, mint). I address the taste issue in the next section on the loss of appetite.

Loss of Appetite

"Nausea and vomiting, fatigue, or a buildup of waste products as cancer cells die can cause a loss of appetite. Some chemotherapy drugs can cause temporary changes in taste and smell, which can make food less appetizing. Some people may not want to eat at all, even though they know they need to. This can lead to weight loss and malnutrition. Having good nutrition during and after chemotherapy is important to help you recover from treatment."

I definitely have a loss of appetite periods during my therapy that caused me to drop from my normal weight of 155 pounds to as low as 133 pounds. Early in my disease when I was experiencing significant pain after eating in my abdomen, chest, and back I quickly came to associate eating with pain. An insight from this experience is to avoid creating such negative associations by avoiding foods and beverages that you normally enjoy when they don't taste right. When the side effect diminishes, you can again enjoy these foods as before.

For example, if you enjoy lemonade but lemonade has an off-putting taste during therapy, then refrain from drinking lemonade until a few days after therapy ends when your taste may return to normal. Also, be open to experimenting with different foods and beverages and get to know at what point in your therapy you may be more receptive to these different foods and beverages. Some food items that you didn't prefer before chemotherapy may now taste just fine to you.

I find that the warmth and savory nature of simple soups with saltine crackers is appealing to me when other foods are not. I also learned that beverages like Gatorade® drink may not be appealing to me at different times during therapy whereas flat, room temperature original Coca-Cola® passes the taste test for me pretty much all of the time. I will stir the soda to help remove the carbonation which can cause annoying belching and uncomfortable gas.

As I entered my halfway point in therapy, I was experiencing an increased lack of taste in food – meals were often like eating cardboard. I learned that some condiments could improve the taste, like ketchup and mild salsa. As you can imagine, it can be challenging to "force" a meal that either tastes odd or has no taste. There really isn't a viable option, of course, because you need to maintain weight and energy to survive.

> Although I strive to get the nutrition I need, I really resent the fact that my efforts are also fueling my cancer. Just another injustice over which we have no control.

Nausea and Vomiting

"Nausea and vomiting can start within the first few hours after chemotherapy drugs are given and usually last about 24 hours. However, nausea and vomiting may start more than 24 hours after treatment and last several days (called delayed nausea and vomiting). Some people may have anticipatory nausea after having a few treatments, where they feel nauseated even before treatment is given because they expect to be sick. The health care team can help you manage nausea and vomiting by prescribing anti-nausea drugs. Not all chemotherapy drugs cause nausea and vomiting. Nausea and vomiting are more likely when combinations of chemotherapy drugs are given."

I'm fortunate that neither nausea nor vomiting has been a problem for me. Although everyone can relate to nausea and vomiting, vomiting can be a particular problem for chemotherapy patients because it can contribute to dehydration which has its own potentially serious consequences as I address in Dehydration under the *Bumps in the Road* section.

Anti-nausea drugs are given to me as part of my infusion at the hospital, and I have two different anti-nausea prescriptions that I take during my home infusion. Note that my health care team has recommended that it is best to stay ahead of nausea rather than to treat it after nausea occurs. Consequently, I take these anti-nausea prescriptions even though I don't feel nauseous, and they have been very effective for me.

Diarrhea/Constipation

Diarrhea and constipation can occur because chemotherapy drugs often affect the cells that line the gastrointestinal (GI) tract. Many factors increase the risk of diarrhea/constipation, including the type and dose of chemotherapy. Diarrhea is often worse when combinations of chemotherapy drugs are given, and both can occur soon after chemotherapy starts and may continue after treatment has ended.

To ensure that I counter the constipation effects of chemotherapy on my GI tract I generally use both Miralax in the morning and Sennokot-S in the evening as required per the advice of my health care team. I also have Immodium® (*loperamide*) handy should diarrhea occur. Other patients note that drugs such as Lomotil (the generic form of diphenoxylate atropine) taken prophylactically before the onset of symptoms may also be effective.

My team recommends that I adjust the use and dose of these products to avoid both diarrhea and constipation. While there is no strict formula for how much of these products to use, over time I've managed by trial and error to make the necessary adjustments.

Thinking and Memory Changes

"Chemotherapy can cause you to have trouble thinking clearly and concentrating. This is often called 'chemo brain.' These effects can go away after chemotherapy is finished or may last up to a year after treatment is over. Sometimes these effects happen long after treatment is finished. Your health care team can suggest ways to help improve concentration and manage changes in memory. They may suggest cognitive exercises that help retrain memory and improve concentration."

I've definitely experienced *chemo brain*.[36] Over my career, I was typically involved in problem-solving that required critical and systems thinking skills. Particularly *thorny* problems required me to take in large amounts of information that I would methodically analyze and synthesize into practical solutions. My cognitive skills are affected during therapy, even after the chemotherapy clears my body.

For example, I had been working on a comprehensive personal financial planning tool that I built in Excel before my diagnosis. This workbook enabled me to input annual gross income, calculate federal and state taxes for net income, input annual expenses, and calculate our net profit/loss. It also tracked investments and used a routine I wrote in Microsoft Visual Basic for Applications (VBA) to estimate probable future returns on investments. The spreadsheet extended its estimates well into the future, providing best- and worst-case outcomes. I honestly can't maintain the spreadsheet at this time due to my chemo brain.

Chemo brain has also affected my ability and desire to read as I once did. I find that I occasionally need to re-read sections to ensure that I properly understand. I ask Diane the same questions she's already answered because I'm not sure if I asked them in the first place. I stopped driving early in my therapy because I didn't trust myself to make good judgments or react quickly. Diane has become my chauffeur – which I learned is pretty easy to get used to.

Low Blood Cell Counts

"Low blood cell counts happen because of chemotherapy's effect on blood cells made in the bone marrow. Blood cell counts often reach their lowest level about 7 to 14 days after chemotherapy. Low blood cell counts are the most common and most serious side effect of chemotherapy. When it happens, the dose of chemotherapy is adjusted right away, or chemotherapy may have to be stopped temporarily. A low white blood cell count (neutropenia or leukopenia) increases the risk for infection. A low platelet count (thrombocytopenia) increases the risk for bruising and bleeding. A low red blood cell count (anemia) causes fatigue, paleness, dizziness, shortness of breath and malaise."

I have experienced low blood cell counts during my therapy; in one instance my white blood count was low enough to postpone the start of a therapy cycle by one week. My health care team added to my therapy an injection of a drug that *nudges* my bone marrow to produce cells. I receive this injection a couple of days after the home infusion pump is removed.

Hair loss

"Hair loss (*alopecia*) is a common side effect of many, but not all, chemotherapy drugs. Hair follicles are damaged by chemotherapy because the drugs affect cells that are growing quickly. It's hard to predict how much hair you will lose and how long hair loss will last because it depends on the type and dose of drugs used as well as your body. Hair loss can happen on any part of the body, not just your head. You may begin to lose hair within a few days or 2 to 3 weeks after chemotherapy starts. Hair usually grows back once you finish chemotherapy."

Initially, I didn't think that the chemotherapy was affecting my hair. Mother Nature was already at work before the chemotherapy started, having turned my hair white and lightening the hair follicle density on the top of my head. However, as I neared the halfway point of my treatments, I noticed that my chemotherapy was rapidly giving Mother Nature a hand by further harvesting my hair. My facial hair, which I used to shave daily, now grows in a very light stubble that easily gives way to even a used razor. My eyebrows, however, continue to grow and require grooming. Go figure.

I understand that hair loss for female cancer patients can be particularly anguishing, and I accept that many men may also lament the effect that hair loss has on their sense of self. For me, hair loss hasn't been an issue. I've considered that I may want to get a very close buzz cut if not a fully shorn head, depending on how much more hair loss I experience. I just hope that my bald head is as attractively shaped as Yul Brenner's, Dwayne Johnson's, or my cousin Randy's.

Sore Mouth

"A sore mouth (also called *stomatitis* or *oral mucositis*) happens because of chemotherapy's effect on cells inside the mouth. Many drugs can cause a sore mouth, but it happens more often when higher doses of drugs are used. Your mouth may become sore anywhere from 5 to 10 days after chemotherapy starts. It often gets better on its own a few weeks after treatment is finished."

"You may develop painful sores, ulcers or infection in the mouth, throat, or gums. Regular mouth care can help prevent a sore mouth and lower the chance of infection. The health care team will tell you how often to clean and rinse your mouth and what to use. Some people may need to take pain medicines."

According to Steven Merlin, "Symptoms of oral mucositis can be ameliorated with an oral rinse especially formulated to address uncomfortable mouth sores (e.g., "Magic Mouthwash"[37]). To address oral thrush[38], the anti-fungal Nystatin[39] may be used; an antibiotic may be used to prevent/treat bacterial infections. For discomfort, Lidocaine or other numbing medication can provide soothing relief. Antihistamines or steroids reduce inflammation and an antacid in a glycerin solution helps to coat the oral mucosa."

Steven also notes "Chemo can reduce the production of saliva which has a bacteriostatic effect protecting teeth. Dry mouth particularly during the overnight hours results in significant bacterial growth. This acts upon the enamel and more vulnerable areas of teeth, particularly areas exposed as a result of receding gums. Often referred to as *Chemo Caries*, it is characterized by a much faster rate of deterioration than normal cavity progression. To promote the production of saliva, some dentists recommend a product called XyliMelts. They are disks placed on the upper gums which adhere and slowly dissolve as they stimulate saliva products. The tabs last about 7 hours." See https://www.oracoat.com/xylimelts.html

A further recommendation from Steven, "Another product to help with the dry mouth during the day is Bioténe. It is a glycerin-based solution that costs the oral mucosa and retains moisture and also stimulates saliva. Rinsing is required throughout the day to maintain protective effects." See https://www.biotene.com/dry-mouth-products/mouthwash/

Finally, Steven observes that "Basic oral hygiene of more frequent brushing, rinsing, flossing and the use of products like GUM Proxibrush for more efficient cleaning between the teeth will help prevent tooth decay." See https://www.gumbrand.com/new-proxabrush.html

Steven suggests that "Chemo patients may want to consider having dental cleanings and check-ups three or four times a year. If dental work is required while on chemo, dentists will prescribe antibiotics for prophylactic use. Cancer patients have an increase of dental issues during as well as long after chemo is completed. Therefore, it is better to see a dental hygienist and dentist on a more frequent basis."

So far, mouth sores haven't been a problem for me. I do have a sensation of something in the back of my throat (like a lump of sand) during infusion periods. I am also sensitive to cold beverages during and shortly after infusions and so drink beverages at room temperature. I occasionally notice a sensitivity inside of my mouth and on my lips, and I use lip balm when my lips feel dry. As I approached the halfway mark of my therapy, I did notice a numbness/tingling in my mouth, lips, and tongue. My teeth also felt numb and that something had become lodged between my teeth even though flossing revealed that nothing was wedged. Go figure.

Difficult or Painful Swallowing, Heartburn, or Pain in the Upper Abdomen

"Pain caused by an inflamed esophagus (called *esophagitis*) can affect eating. You may need to change what you eat or take pain-relieving medicines if you have trouble swallowing or it hurts to swallow."

Part of my daily routine includes a 24-hour Nexium® pill in the morning which seems to keep indigestion at bay. During infusion periods I have experienced the sensation that something is "stuck" in the back of my throat. Cough drops or drinking something warm seems to relieve this sensation. I've also gotten some relief by gargling with salt water.

Skin Changes

"Some drugs can cause skin problems or skin irritation. Skin changes can happen during and for some time after chemotherapy. Skin reactions can include redness, itching, dryness, rash, or nail changes. Skin may also be more sensitive to or easily irritated by the sun during chemotherapy treatment."

Steven Merlin notes, "Sensitivity to the sun may develop as a result of chemotherapy. Often a memory response occurs in an area where one experienced sunburn earlier in life. A reaction to sun exposure known as heat urticaria produces a tingling sensation, rash as a result of histamine being released by mast cells in the skin, and more intense sunburn in the same area."

So far, I've noticed three changes related to my skin. First, my normally oily skin is now clear but not dry. Second, a small patch of chronic dry skin I had on one of my eyelids has disappeared. Third, sagging skin due to my weight and muscle loss. I use CeraVe® moisturizing cream[40] on my feet after showering. CeraVe is readily absorbed into my skin and does not have the greasy feeling of some moisturizers. The result has been very positive, yielding softer skin without cracks and flakes. Other patients recommend Keri® lotion which is also non-greasy and readily absorbed in the skin.

Eye Changes

"Some chemotherapy drugs cause eye changes, such as blurry vision, watery eyes and trouble wearing contact lenses. Tell the doctor or health care team if you have changes to your eyes."

So far, I haven't experienced specific eye problems like blurring or double vision. I have noticed that I may not be focusing as before, and that may be due in part to the time I spend on my mobile phone and computer screen. Before my chemotherapy began, I did experience dry eye that I managed with eye drops like Systane® and Refresh® Plus which do seem to help during chemotherapy also.

Pain

"Some chemotherapy drugs can cause painful side effects, such as aching in the muscles and joints, headaches, and stomach pains. Pain may be felt as burning, numbness, tingling or shooting pains in the hands and feet (called peripheral nerve damage). This type of pain can last long after treatment ends. The health care team will tell you what medicines to use to relieve the pain."

I haven't yet experienced pain except in isolated cases (e.g., the chest pain I describe under Bumps in the Road). I have also experienced occasional numbness and high sensitivity to cold in my fingers during chemotherapy.

> Previous to my cancer diagnosis I had occasionally exhibited Raynaud's phenomenon[41], numbness of the fingers in response to cold temperatures or stress that restricts blood flow and turns the digits white.[42] On one

occasion shortly after infusions, I reached into the freezer to retrieve a bag of frozen vegetables, and immediately my fingertips felt like I had touched a red-hot poker. Wearing a pair of oven gloves will provide you with effective protection from this cold hypersensitivity and pain. Other patients recommend glove liners, wool-lined mittens, and battery-powered electric gloves for use in the winter season.

In addition to the Canadian Cancer Society (CCS) list of common side effects stated above, I've also experienced the following.

Weight Loss

Weight loss is not necessarily due solely to the therapy and likely includes cancer that is interfering with my ability to digest food. The therapy certainly curbs my appetite as certain foods don't taste right during my therapy and until the chemotherapy clears my body. So, consuming enough calories to maintain and hopefully gain weight requires that I eat not for pleasure but for survival.

During therapy, I tend to favor salty soups and certain sweets like pies and French toast with plenty of maple syrup. I do occasionally drink caloric supplements like Boost, but at times the viscous nature of Boost isn't something that I particularly enjoy and can force, especially if I feel full of other food that I've eaten before drinking Boost. Note that as the chemotherapy clears my body my appetite does slowly return, and I find that I can eat a larger selection and amount of food.

Steven Merlin notes that "Enterade®, a protein supplement, may be more appealing than Boost and Ensure (https://enterade.com). Enterade currently comes in two flavors and is being recommended by an increasing number of chemotherapy clinics. A list of protein supplements can be found at https://maxhealthliving.com/meal-replacement-shakes-for-cancer-patients/"

There is a certain *oddity* to my unintentional weight loss. I had struggled with obesity in my youth, weighing in at a bit over 250 pounds when a senior in high school (this on a 5' 6" frame). My pants were a men's waist size of 46" or

48" that had to be severely tailored to shorten the length of the pant to fit me. Although the pants were of good quality, the rubbing of my hefty thighs regularly created holes in the abused material.

In my senior year, I joined the wrestling team as a heavyweight (I honestly can't say why I joined the team). Although the various wrestling maneuvers and hours of relentless drills were a challenge for an overweight kid with no prior physical conditioning, I managed to have a successful junior varsity season while losing weight and gaining strength and confidence.

My weight struggle continued over the years after high school until I finally got my mind right and my weight stable at about 155 pounds. My cancer achieved weight loss in just a few weeks which was much faster than what I could attain in months of dieting and exercise.

Now I eat foods that I avoided like COVID-19 before my diagnosis to help maintain my weight: cinnamon buns, pies, mac and cheese, regular Coke, etc. Even with these high-calorie selections, however, I barely maintain my abnormally low body weight. Weight gain during cancer is just another of those many things over which I seem to have little control.

By the way, although you may be struggling to maintain or increase weight, it's also important to get some kind of regular exercise. On days when I can't walk Ozzie, I will pace inside the house or on our patio. I also do *high knees* where I balance myself with palms on a wall and then repeatedly lift my knees at least to my waist if possible[43].

Chair squats are also a beneficial exercise to help maintain large muscle tone. This exercise is done by sitting in a chair and then repeatedly rising from the chair and returning to the chair again without using your arms for support[44].

Finally, I occasionally use exercise bands for my biceps[45] and chest muscles. Note that you can purchase an inexpensive exercise band kit that includes hardware that temporarily attaches to a door, but you can also simply wrap the exercise band around your shoulders[46]. Exercise bands offer the benefits of compactness, lightweight, a constant force, and no worries about dropping a dumbbell on your foot or the cat!

Feeling Cold

Not to be confused with fever chills, I occasionally feel cold in environments where others are comfortable. I suspect that my weight loss and blood counts may have something to do with this effect. My simple solutions include a long-sleeve shirt, a lightweight blanket, and moving from air conditioning to a seat outside in the sun as the weather permits.

Hand Tremors

Hand tremors tend to occur in me during infusion periods and until the chemotherapy clears my body. When these tremors are occurring, I may drop items and find simple coordination practically impossible (e.g., writing clearly). Tremors force me to use two hands to hold a cup to my lips and make it nearly impossible for me to get the blade of a small screwdriver into the screw slot and to keep it there as I tighten the screw. The tremors normally stop on Days 4-5.

Misreading My Gut

Because of the effect that chemotherapy has on the GI system, I find that I can't always understand what my gut is trying to tell me. Sometimes I have a hollow feeling that may suggest I'm hungry or something else. At times my gut gurgles which may signal normal gut motility, gas, or something else. I just try to go with the flow until the sensations work their way out.

Upset Stomach

Not nausea, rather more of a *belly ache* that comes and goes. I've tried antacids like Tums® which weren't very effective, and anti-gas products like Gas-X® that seem to help if the source of the ache is bloating. Alka-Seltzer® seems to be reliably effective for me, possibly because it includes aspirin which is an anti-inflammatory.

Bumps in the Road

Although my therapy has gone ahead much as my health care team anticipated, I have encountered several unforeseen events that I describe below.

Dehydration

I've never been one to drink the recommended eight cups of water a day. I marvel at how some associates and family are constantly sipping from a large water bottle throughout the day and I wonder if they are part fish and why they don't explode with all of that liquid in their guts.

This reluctance to drown myself daily has led to problems in the past. For example, I have experienced crippling back spasms over the years, a couple of which landed me in the ER. During these periods my low level of hydration likely only made the problem worse, causing me to faint.

Early in my therapy, I had a fainting episode that collapsed me in the bathroom, bouncing my head off the tile floor. Fortunately, Diane heard the thump and was assessing me moments later. During this event, I was cold and shaking uncontrollably and had difficulty speaking loudly enough for Diane to hear my answers to her questions.

Diane called EMS and got assistance from a neighbor to help wrangle Ozzie and prep for the arrival of the ambulance. I was so weak that I relied almost entirely on the strength of the EMS personnel to get me off the floor and onto a stretcher for transport. At the hospital, I was given fluids to rehydrate and a CT scan to confirm that I didn't have head trauma from my fall. Some hours were consumed from the time of my collapse until I returned home. It could have been a lot worse.

The takeaway from this story is to avoid dehydration at all costs. Even if you don't feel like drinking, make the effort. If one beverage isn't palatable to you then try others. For me, sometimes Gatorade® or lemonade are good ways to keep hydrated, while other times I rely on flat Coca-Cola® or plain water. My sense of taste changes and I have to switch between beverages.

Another way I try to manage hydration is to eat foods that have high fluid content. I eat a lot of soup during those times when I'm not inclined to eat or drink. I will also cook plain ramen noodles in broth, avoiding the chemical-rich flavor packages included in some products. Other foods I include in my diet are granola with milk, oatmeal made with additional water or milk, canned fruit with juice, and chunks of watermelon. I've also made a *melon sauce* by blending chunks of cantaloupe with a little water until it has the consistency of applesauce. Granola in particular can provide a lot of calories in a relatively small volume which may help with digestion and avoid a bloated feeling.

Bile Duct Obstruction

As I described earlier, the liver and pancreas work together to provide proper digestion of food we eat (among other functions). The substances produced by the liver and pancreas travel through ducts into the intestines. When these ducts become obstructed, serious problems can occur such as a backup of bile in the liver that can cause organ failure.

One of the first questions that my health care team asked me in my very first meetings was the color of my urine and stool, specifically, was my urine dark or my stool lightly colored like clay? I understood the dark urine concern, as that's one of the signs of dehydration, but the stool color concern was new to me. Turns out that when a bile duct obstruction occurs a telltale sign is a lightening of stool color.

This event started one morning when I noticed that my urine had gotten as dark as strongly brewed tea and that my stool was clay-colored. This change alerted Diane who contacted my health care team, and my health care team arranged for me to get to the hospital as soon as possible to diagnose what was going on and to take any necessary intervention.

The tumor on my pancreas is located atop a major vein and very near my bile duct. Apparently, the tumor was encroaching on the duct, creating an obstruction that would need to be corrected. My physicians decided to perform an Endoscopic Retrograde Cholangiopancreatography (ERCP) (described under the Upper Endoscopy section).

For my procedure a small, flexible tube (*stent*) was inserted into the obstructed part of the bile duct, forcing it open. Performed under anesthesia, the procedure was relatively quick, and I felt no pain afterward. The effects of the stent were rapid, and the color of my urine and stool quickly returned to normal.

If we had hesitated to bring the color change to the attention of my health care team, the outcome could have been much worse. **Always keep your health care team in the loop when things change, especially if the team forewarned you to look for specific changes**.

A Hospital Stay

I was admitted to the hospital for the ERCP procedure described above and had a couple of nights' stay at the hospital. If you've never had a hospital stay, then you may find the experience a hodgepodge of emotions.

You may be bored much of the time during a hospital stay because you are pretty much restricted to your room and bed. You will likely have a television, a chair for visitors, and a bathroom, but other "home comforts" will be absent. We tend to become complacent about our normal environment and may not appreciate the luxuries of our own bed, refrigerator, favorite chair, and so forth.

Due to my fatigue, low energy level, and "fall risk" designation, I spent most of my time in bed. If I needed to use the toilet, then I would have to ring a nurse for help. Initially, a small plastic urinal while I stood at the side of the bed under nurse supervision was required. For a private person like me who also values his independence, this situation was not pleasant, and I was happy when I was able to use the toilet independently with only nursing assistance to get me into and out of the bathroom.

You may also be exhausted because of the round-the-clock routine of a hospital. During a hospital stay, you are regularly checked in on by nursing staff who document your progress, administer medications as needed, and ensure a smooth hand-off to other nurses as shifts change. Other health care professionals will also visit to take vital signs like heart rate and blood pressure, administer EKG and other prescribed diagnostic tests, and help with care issues like personal hygiene.

Returning home after a hospital stay is like returning to the United States after an international trip. You may have been well cared for during your trip and learned new things about different cultures, but you also are reminded as was Dorothy in *The Wizard of Oz* that there's no place like home, there's no place like home…

Chest Pain

When I'm feeling well, I try to increase the amount of food that I eat during a meal. This can be a fine balancing act, eating more without creating the feeling of being bloated which kills my appetite. It was during one of these more normal meals that I may have gone one bite too far.

Everything was fine immediately after the meal; however, things quickly changed, and for the worst when I suddenly felt a sharp pain in the center of my chest. Imagine that someone decided to hammer a steel rod into your breastbone and through your back and you have an idea of the deep, penetrating, and unrelenting pain I experienced. With every moment, the pain became more intense, and lying down didn't do anything to help resolve the pain. It is one of the few times in my life that Diane could recall when I was moaning in pain.

Diane wanted to call EMS again and I (unreasonably) wanted to wait a bit to see if the pain would subside. Diane administered a morphine prescription that I had been given – a drug that I didn't think I would ever need, and that seemed to slowly reduce the intensity of the pain. More settled under the influence of morphine, I was open to reason and agreed that a trip to the ER was a good idea.

Rather than taking me to the local ER, Diane decided to drive 30-minutes to the ER at Duke Hospital in Durham. Duke physicians were managing my care there, and if something serious were uncovered, then I would be in the right place at the right time.

Making one's way from the ER receiving area to a treatment room in a busy ER is a challenge that you can only understand by experiencing it yourself. The receiving area may be large but often not large enough to accommodate the number of patients seeking help. Patients include people from all levels of society, many in clear distress, but whose issues are not as potentially life-threatening as others who have come for assistance (e.g., trauma, heart attack). Thanks to Diane's crisp explanation of my situation, the ER staff had me immediately moved to a treatment room where I could be monitored until a physician was available.

The staff was swamped that evening and so I was on monitoring for several hours until an assessment could be made. A chest x-ray and EKG were ordered to help ensure that there wasn't anything abnormal in my heart (a potential side effect of some chemotherapy drugs). The results did not show any cardiac or other problems that might have created the chest pain. The origin of the pain was deemed unrelated to my earlier meal and likely related to the bile duct stent that I had received. Whatever the reason I was happy that the pain was gone.

I don't recall exactly when Diane and I arrived at the ER that evening, but we weren't discharged until sometime around 4:30 the following morning – and Diane had to work that day.

PATIENT PORTALS

Online and mobile app patient portals can offer significant benefits to you and your caregivers during your therapy. These patient portals are efficient ways to connect directly with your health care team on questions or concerns you may have, to be reminded of appointments, and to check in before going to the hospital. I **highly recommend** that you take the time to get onto both an online and mobile patient portal app if available to you. At the same time, I've seen what I feel are performance inefficiencies in these platforms.

For example, some of the check-in questions are to confirm information that may reasonably change, e.g., is the visit due to an accident, are you coming to your appointment from your home or another facility, have you fallen within the last 30 days, and do you have any special needs (like a wheelchair). At the same time, I witness what appears to me to be redundant and inefficient behaviors.

For example, I'm on Medicare which requires that I confirm, during **every check-in,** if I'm receiving Black Lung (BL) benefits, if my care will be paid by a government research program, if I'm entitled to benefits through the Department of Veterans Affairs (DVA), if my illness was due to a work-related accident/condition. I also have secondary Medicare coverage for which I confirm, during **every check-in,** if I have end-stage renal disease, if I'm currently employed or the date of my retirement, if my spouse is currently employed and the name and address of her employer, and if I have coverage under your spouse's group health plan (GHP).

I've had the experience where I checked in via my patient portal at home, but still had to answer the same questions when I arrived at the facility – shouldn't that information be immediately available thanks to my online check-in? On at least one occasion, I was asked the same set of questions in two different departments in one day (morning and afternoon). How likely is it that most of my previous answers would change; for example, the employment status for me or Diane, if I have black lung or end-stage renal disease, or from where I arrived for my appointment?

For some reason, we were regularly asked if Diane was still working and her employer. Although we watched as the admitting personnel updated that information, it didn't seem to "stick" in the database. I acknowledge that none of these quirks in any way impact my care, rather they can just add an unnecessary annoyance to a hospital visit, especially on those days when I'm not feeling very well.

During my business career, I have worked on process improvement like those that business analysts are regularly tasked to tackle. It seems to me that some of the patient portal issues I relay above could benefit from a few relatively simple updates in how they perform. If you encounter these kinds of odd portal behaviors that I described above, then you ought to let the hospital know about them so they can try to improve (or explain) their procedures.

Note that telling the person entering the data won't make any difference, they are just doing their job and are not able to make any changes to the platform. If the hospital sends a performance survey, then that would be a good way to share your observations. You could also write a letter to the IT department of the hospital and ask them to pass your comments to the parties who maintain the platform.

> **Note** that patient portals may advise you about lab blood work and procedures immediately after a health care professional enters test and procedure information. These results can be confusing and misleading to those who lack a medical background.

For example, just because some blood measurements fall outside of the "normal" range does not necessarily indicate a problem. Rather it is the interpretation made by a physician regarding all of the blood measurements and other diagnostic information that helps create a complete diagnostic picture. Similarly, medical terminology regarding procedures like CT scans requires specific medical expertise for correct interpretation.

Never "play doctor" by trying to interpret test and procedure results or by consulting "Dr. Google." **Always** speak with your health care team about the meaning of tests and procedures as they pertain to your health and care.

****

Now that we've finished much of the main nuts-and-bolts *explanatory* sections on cancer, procedures, and my personal journey, let's move on to the more *meditative* aspects of this book.

I'm providing these meditative sections to establish a foundation for the final section of the book where I explain how I'm dealing with my disease. Without knowing how I view the world; you may not understand how my worldview drives my thoughts and actions. Likewise, your worldview will certainly affect how you approach your diagnosis, therapy, and prognosis.

EMOTIONAL, RELIGIOUS, AND PHILOSOPHICAL PERSPECTIVES

Seeking the "meaning" of your cancer diagnosis and prognosis opens wide the doors to emotional, religious, and philosophical considerations. These contemplations will affect not only you but also your family and friends who care about you and want to do whatever they can to help. In this section, I share my experiences and thoughts on emotional, religious, and philosophical aspects.

I don't offer my comments to challenge your beliefs or to attempt to influence you in any way. My goal here is to explain how I view the world which may be very different from the way that you view the world. I'm not looking for an argument or debate. I simply hope that my views may offer some thought-provoking ideas that you hadn't considered, and which may be helpful to you, your family, and your friends.

Emotional Perspectives

When I refer to emotional events, I mean those times that cause an automatic, unthinking reaction in us. The way we feel the first time that someone tells us they love us, when a spouse asks for a divorce, when a promotion isn't given, when a loyal and gravely ill canine companion needs to be euthanized. Emotional responses are often the result of expectations unfulfilled – when something that we had fully expected to happen, didn't.

Working our way through our own emotional feelings can be a grueling experience, rich in second-guessing, fault-finding, and resentment. When others are involved in a shared event that involvement can create an emotional reaction in them, too. In this situation, the experiences of the patient and others become intertwined and more complex. It's not just about resolving our own emotional issues, but also understanding how others around us – like family and friends, are managing their emotions.

When Diane and I got my diagnosis, we both had an emotional response. Our responses, however, were different. I was surprisingly calm – perhaps too calm given the situation. Diane put up a strong front but was clearly struggling and one afternoon she was unable to keep it in any longer.

We were sitting on our patio, and I was running a finger along my forearm, examining its features in the sunlight. Due to my weight loss, my skin was sagging, and my veins appeared like a network of blue pipe work just below the surface. I didn't notice that Diane was watching me until I heard her weeping. I asked her what was wrong, and she replied, "I ache for you."

I put my hand on her shoulder and told her, "It's okay," meaning that I felt I was dealing with the situation well and she didn't need to worry about me. At that moment it started to dawn on me that although the cancer diagnosis was mine, we both would be affected albeit in different ways. I realized that I needed to adopt a more open attitude, listen more, and talk less. I needed to hear not only the words that Diane was saying but their meaning. I needed to look for avenues where I could embrace and express empathy for what she was experiencing.

We spoke further about her concerns and fears which included her feeling of helplessness and also how she would go on after my passing. Part of our discussion was on support resources that were available to us either through Duke Hospital or independently. These resources included both group therapy sessions and one-on-one sessions with a therapist.

I told Diane that I wasn't interested in group sessions with other cancer patients. I reasoned that I had reached a position where I was ready to embrace therapy and accepting of whatever outcome occurred. Diane is a more outgoing person and so decided to try a group session which revealed an interesting insight to her.

The group session that Diane attended did not include any people with a clinical background – no nurses, physicians, or other health care workers. Diane learned from her experience that she could not step out of her clinician role, and so she found herself wanting to offer advice as she did in navigating the care for her patients. Diane needed to talk to someone who could do for her what she does for the families of her patients, and no one in the group that she attended had the experience or skill to do so.

Recognizing that some form of therapy would be beneficial, Diane turned to a psychologist whom she knew to arrange one-on-one counseling with us. These sessions were conducted over Zoom and lasted an hour each. During the session, the therapist would ask open-ended questions that were intended to get us talking about how my diagnosis was affecting us. These questions also encouraged us to speak plainly and understand what we each needed on an emotional level.

I had decided at the time of my diagnosis that I would refrain from any argument or debate about my treatment. I promised Diane that I would faithfully follow the advice of both my medical team in general and her guidance on what I needed to do on a day-to-day basis. Likewise, I tried to approach our therapy sessions with openness and deference. What made this goal for therapy a bit of a challenge for me was my on-again, off-again view of the power of psychological therapy.

Trained in the "hard sciences" I didn't hold "soft sciences" like psychology in high regard in my college years. It was only later as I approached my 40s that I turned to therapy to help me through a challenging time that included a job loss, a divorce, a home sale, and a relocation. I realized that I needed help and worked with a therapist. I learned that being able to speak openly about what I was thinking exposed unreasonable fears I held and false presumptions I had made.

During our sessions with the therapist, I tried to accept anything said as a true and important issue even if a statement didn't make sense to me at the time. I learned that Diane needed to feel closer to me and that my declarations to her that I was okay were not giving her the emotional assurances that she was seeking. I promised to be more open with her and shared how I was dealing with my diagnosis and prognosis so she would know that I wasn't intentionally closed emotionally.

After several sessions, we both felt that our communications had become more open and transparent. My diagnosis and course of therapy would continue as before, but how Diane and I approached the challenges was more coordinated and empowering. Of course, Diane and I are human and so we may occasionally miss a beat, but overall, I feel that the therapy has been helpful to us.

If you haven't yet found some form of psychological support, either in group sessions or one-to-one with a reliable therapist, then I encourage you to do so sooner than later.

Family and Friends

In addition to your own emotional needs and the needs of a spouse or significant other, there are the emotional needs of family and friends. Those near and dear to you want to help in any way that they can from lending a hand to make your life easier, to offering an ear if you need to rage against your disease or are seeking encouragement. For a private and (normally) independent person like myself, accepting offers of help can be difficult because it *signals* that I'm somehow lacking the capacity to handle myself. Of course, this signaling is my perception and not necessarily what those offering help mean to convey. Being attentive to what people are offering and being open to their largess can go a long way to serving the emotional needs of those around us.

For example, when the wife of a neighbor learned of my diagnosis, she delivered a delicious dish to us for dinner one night. When she returned to pick up her serving plate, she spoke about different desserts that she had made. I listened politely but didn't respond to any of her descriptions. What I had missed, of course, was that she was trying to find out what kind of dessert she could make for me. Had I been paying closer attention, then I may have suggested that one of the desserts sounded delicious and she would have happily created the dish for us as another expression of support. Truly listening is a skill worth developing.

My mother and brothers likewise offered their help and support. My brothers pressed to come down to stay with us and lend a hand. My mother wanted to visit and see me in person. Living in Pennsylvania, however, my mother and brothers are easily a seven to twelve-hour drive away from our home in North Carolina, depending on traffic.

Further, our son Tom, a remote IT worker, had moved from California to our home so he could help manage the house and provide emotional support for Diane. We had set up an office with a bed for

Tom. I was already using a bedroom separate from the master bedroom that Diane used so there was no space to accommodate additional on-site help.

Even a simple visit offered its own challenges. My mother is in her nineties, and although she is in remarkable health, a long drive would be difficult for her. Flights would be difficult, too, due to the somewhat isolated location of my mother's home, and also because of COVID exposure concerns for her.

Likewise, a drive to my mother's home could be difficult for me depending on when in my two-week therapy cycle the trip could be scheduled. At my mother's house I would not be near a major hospital should I need medical assistance. One of my brothers lives in Philadelphia, a couple of hours closer to me, and perhaps his home could be a meeting place. It would be a much shorter drive for my mother and if I needed medical assistance, then I would be close to several renowned Philadelphia hospitals.

Rather than attempt any of these live visits, however, we decided to try Zoom calls on those alternating weeks when the chemotherapy had washed out and I would regain my strength and focus. Although not the same as sitting around a table with my family, the ability for the family to see me and for me to see their reactions during our conversations turned out to be a very good thing.

If you, your family, and your friends have access to the internet and a Zoom account, then I would urge you to try this communication method. If you have the necessary computer hardware and internet connection but not a Zoom account, then you can sign up for a free Zoom account (see https://zoom.us/pricing). The free account limits call time to 40 minutes which is sufficient for a quick catch-up.

Of course, there are other electronic means of communication like email and text messaging, both of which I use to stay in touch nearly every day with a few old friends. One friend and I rely upon text messages but occasionally we have a short phone call for a live, interactive chat.

You may also want to consider a traditional letter sent through the US Postal Service. There is something about putting pen to paper to share your thoughts with others. Doing so affords you a quiet time to collect and record your thoughts. The addressee of your letter receives something unique to you – your hand-written script, in an ink color and on stationary that you selected. Written letters are more durable than communications in the digital world, and you and your recipients may choose to store the messages in a nice keepsake box.[47]

A Note to Family and Friends

> This section is for those families and friends who are reading this book. Above, I offer advice on how the cancer patient can be receptive to your desire to help and address your emotional needs. It's also important that you consider how your well-intentioned words and actions can affect the patient in ways you do not intend. You can do this by reminding yourself that the cancer patient is living in a kind of parallel universe.

In our early meetings with my health care team, they provided Diane and me with some insight into what I might expect from the disease, therapy, and side effects. I also went looking for information from other reputable sources like Mayo Clinic and the Centers for Disease Control and Prevention (CDC). I imagined what it would be like when I was fully in the life of a cancer patient – what I would experience and how I would react. Once I was in the disease, however, I quickly learned how poorly my imagination foresaw my reality.

On the outside, both the cancer patient and those around her seem to move in the same world, bathing in the same sunlight, eating the same food, and listening to the same music. However, the cancer patient's experience includes chemo brain, fatigue, emotional swings, loss of appetite, and other challenges that must be lived to be truly understood. What you may imagine the cancer patient is experiencing is likely as wrong as were my own early speculations. What might seem like a commonsense suggestion that you make to the cancer patient, may make about as much sense to the patient as speaking to her in a foreign language that she does not know.

I have in mind, for example, how your offers to help might need to be paced so the patient doesn't feel overwhelmed or pressured to do something that they don't want to do. If you find yourself constantly asking how the patient is feeling, or if you can do such-and-so for them, then you might want to back off for a while. As I noted above, learning to truly listen is a skill well worth developing.

Likewise, if the patient wants to do something by themselves, like tending to a garden, another home project, or shopping, then I would urge you to let her do so. Pressing the patient to let you do these sorts of things for them may make the patient feel inadequate and weak. These feelings may suggest to the patient that she's dealing poorly with a serious disease and that the disease is in control. You can help the patient by creating some room to maneuver and to have some basic independence.

By establishing an open channel of communication between you and the patient, the patient knows that they can rely upon your help when they need it, and you can be assured that they will ask for help when the time is right.

Religious Perspectives

Religion plays an important role in the lives of many people around the globe. The Central Intelligence Agency (CIA) World Factbook[48] offers interesting insights into the predominance of religions by geographical area, and Pew Research Center regularly offers great insights into Religion in America.[49]

Because religion influences our views of both the temporal world and the possibility of an afterlife, it's understandable that religion also colors how we respond to news like a cancer diagnosis and prognosis. Speculating about how you will deal with your mortality when you are healthy isn't the same as actually facing your mortality when you have a life-threatening disease. Living with cancer forces you to reexamine how you thought you would respond to mortality questions versus how you are actually responding. Some may look to religion (or philosophy) to find answers to the many questions that a cancer diagnosis raises like:

- Why did I get cancer although I was relatively healthy otherwise, a non-smoker and teetotaler who watches my weight and exercises?
- Why did I get cancer when others I know who are lifetime smokers, drinkers, and overweight seem to be doing just fine?
- What did I do "wrong" and why am I being "punished?"

In this section, I discuss my own religious background and current thinking. I note that this section is lengthier than the sections on Emotional and Philosophical Perspectives. Given the role of religion in my life, however, I feel it's important to provide the background to you below so you can compare it to your own experience with religion. Again, I am **not** trying to challenge anyone's religious belief or to convert anyone to my way of thinking. Rather, I hope to provide a foundation for the last section of this book, Wrapping it Up.

When I refer to religion, I'm speaking specifically of *formal* religions that adhere to "a specific fundamental set of beliefs and practices generally agreed upon by a number of persons or sects" and "the practice of religious beliefs; ritual observance of faith."[50] These formal religions typically have a key spiritual leader, "an authoritative list of books accepted as Holy Scripture" (a *canon*), and a physical place where the faithful congregate (churches, synagogues, mosques, etc.). My religious experience is as a Roman Catholic, raised in a small Pennsylvania coal-mining town during the 1950s and into the 1970s.

I feel it's important to stipulate the location and time frame above because culture impacts the interpretation of basic religious teachings and practices. A Roman Catholic from a small Pennsylvania coal-mining town does not have the same context as the Kennedy Compound in Hyannis Port, Massachusetts. Further, Catholicism, as was taught and practiced in mid-nineteenth century America, is likely not the same as Catholicism taught and practiced in Cotonou, Africa today.

My exposure to Roman Catholicism included parochial grade and high school, and two Jesuit universities. As a child, I was trained with the *Baltimore Catechism*[51], a book that provided simple answers to questions of faith that a youngster (or adult) would need. I was also an altar boy, serving while the mass was still conducted in Latin, the priests' backs turned to the faithful much of the time. I continued serving when

English replaced Latin and the priests and altar boys did a 180 to face the congregation most of the time.

I recall my father driving me to mass at six in the morning before starting his daily and lengthy commute to his job. I also took part in Midnight mass at Christmas, processions for the various liturgical holidays, confession, and receiving communion. During Lent, when all the statues were draped in purple[52] and the focus of attention was on the ornate monstrance[53] atop the altar, I would take part in the prayerful devotion of *eucharistic adoration*.[54] All was going as intended by my parents and community on the Faith front – until I went away to college.

In the collegiate setting, I was removed from the *groupthink* of my small town and exposed to a greater variety of people and perspectives. I started to question the years of dogmatic practice that I had followed and to ask myself if my Faith offered me any real value. I was introduced to different religious thought and philosophies, including Taoism which resonated with me (more under Philosophical Perspectives). I currently refer to myself as an *agnostic* – a term that is widely misunderstood by both people of Faith and atheists, and a term that requires some explanation.

As noted above, a person of Faith adheres to a fundamental set of beliefs and practices about one or many gods. By contrast, an atheist is, "a person who does not believe in the existence of a god or any gods."[55] An Agnostic may be defined as "a person who holds the view that any ultimate reality (such as God) is unknown and probably unknowable."

The agnostic position is not one of indecision. Rather the agnostic makes no decision in the absence of proof sources that she finds are reasoned and compelling. If you want to learn more about the origin of the term agnostic and the nature of agnostics, then I recommend you read *What Is an Agnostic* by Bertrand Russell.[56]

No one thing caused me to drift from my Roman Catholic faith toward an agnostic view but rather numerous observations that together moved me. The following are a few of my observations.

Overly Complicated

It seems to me that formal religions start out with a simple premise that becomes more complicated and bureaucratic the longer the religion is sustained. Somehow, the unpretentious story of Jesus and his disciples preaching among the common people has morphed into elaborate churches and real estate, a hierarchy of command and control, fancy robes, a treasure in art, and more. If you aren't familiar with *The Life and Morals of Jesus of Nazareth* (also known as the *Thomas Jefferson Bible)*, then I recommend it to you. According to The Jefferson Bible website,

> *"The Life and Morals of Jesus of Nazareth* was created in 1820 by Thomas Jefferson. He was seventy-seven years old when he constructed his book by cutting excerpts of the New Testament Gospels from six printed volumes published in English, French, Latin and Greek. Jefferson edited and arranged the passages in a chronological order to tell the story of Jesus's life, parables and moral teachings. Jefferson lived in a world where political rulers routinely established a single faith as the official religion. He promoted religious freedom in order to secure the rights of differing religions and to protect the freedom of an individual to practice the religion of their choosing."[57]

Note that the founding fathers did not require that a citizen adheres to any religious belief and that their views on religion were more nuanced than the simplistic claims that some promote today.[58] According to Dr. Gregg Frazer, Professor of History & Political Studies at The Master's University,

> "…both the Christian Right and the secular Left are largely wrong about the religious beliefs of America's key Founders and, consequently, their prescriptions for America based on those assumptions are also wrong. America's Founders were not all Christians, and they did not intend to create a Christian nation." [59]

Remember, too, that Jesus and his disciples were Jews (not Christians) who were viewed by mainstream Judaism as a kind of cult that was at odds with the Jewish orthodoxy. According to biblical accounts, the crucifixion of Jesus was something actively sought by opponents of Jesus' new form of Judaism.

> They cried out, "Away with him, away with him, crucify him!" Pilate said to them, "Shall I crucify your King?" The chief priests answered, "We have no king but Caesar."[60]

I doubt that Jesus would recognize or approve of modern versions of Christianity that have become a new orthodoxy – slow-moving, political, and intransigent. If you are a person of Faith, then think about the full history of your own religion, how it transformed into what it is today, and how that transformation might have degraded and obscured the original meaning of the religion.

Contradictory

I don't recall ever being schooled as a child or at college on the many contradictions in the *Bible* from the punishment of crime to the power of God.[61] Atheists and Agnostics aren't the only ones who point out these contradictions. Bart D. Ehrman, the James A. Gray Distinguished Professor of Religious Studies at the University of North Carolina, Chapel Hill, has written extensively on biblical contradictions.[62]

How can one rely upon the claim that the *Bible*, for example, is the immutable word of God, when the Gospels of Matthew, Mark, Luke, and John were written decades after the actual events, by unknown authors[63], and with inconsistent narratives?[64]

Intransigent

Formal religions set and adhere to their articles of faith, basic beliefs that cannot change whatever contradicting evidence may be provided. This inflexibility is due to the faithful believing that their sacred scripture and dogma rightly express the immutable "word of God" his plans and laws.

A response to those who may challenge the faithful is *apologetics,* a practice that is intended to assure that "the credentials of the Christian religion amply suffice to vindicate the act of faith as a rational act, and to discredit the estrangement of the skeptic and unbeliever as unwarranted and culpable."[65] According to the Christian Research Institute[66],

> "Since Christianity posits a certain knowledge and understanding of God, it is the task of the Christian apologist to demonstrate the grounds of biblical revelation and to establish why placing one's faith in Christianity is not only reasonable but also existentially vital.
>
> Christians have a biblical mandate to engage in apologetics. Peter said, "Always be ready to make a defense to everyone who asks you to give an account for the hope that is in you, yet with gentleness and reverence (1 Pet. 3:15; NASB). The word translated here as "make a defense" is the Greek, apologia.
>
> The apologist par excellence from biblical times was the apostle Paul himself. The *Bible* tells us that Paul "reasoned" with unbelievers in order to explain the truths of Christianity to them. Paul used terms and arguments his contemporary audience could understand, and he provided "reasoned" responses to their objections (e.g., Acts 17:17). Paul instructed others to carry on the apologetic task, saying that we must "demolish arguments and every pretension that sets itself up against the knowledge of God" (2 Corinthians 10:5)."

The *reasoning* referred to by apologists is not the same as reasoning used in the sciences. A key difference is that apologists accept their dogmatic articles of faith as true and unassailable so they cannot change their position even in the presence of strong counterevidence.

By contrast, reasoning in well-done science starts with "a tentative assumption made in order to draw out and test its logical or empirical consequences"[67] (a *hypothesis*) and creates experiments with the assumption that there will be no difference between a baseline and the phenomenon that they are testing (the *null hypothesis*[68]). The researcher determines **in advance of the experiments** what kind of difference would need to be observed in the experiment for a true difference to be revealed. If that difference is not seen, then the hypothesis fails and a new hypothesis is sought. The scientific method has been successfully used to determine, for example, if new drug therapies are more effective than existing drug therapies.

It is only after several hypotheses have been methodically tested by different means and parties that a "scientifically acceptable general principle or body of principles"[69] is accepted as a *theory*. In other words, the dismissive phrase "It's just theory" either naively or intentionally lumps any untested speculation with actual theories.

An enlightening example of this difference between religious and scientific reasoning is an exchange during a debate on Creationism between "the science guy" Bill Nye and Christian fundamentalist Ken Ham.[70,71] When each was asked by the moderator, "What if anything would ever change your mind?"

Ham (who bases his view on the *Bible*) replied (bold mine),

> **"I'm a Christian**. And as a Christian, I can't prove it to you, but God has definitely shown me very clearly through his Word and shown himself in the person of Jesus Christ...And so, as far as the word of God is concerned, **no one's ever going to convince me that the word of God is not true."**

Nye (who bases his view on evidence-based science, replied (bold mine),

> **"We would need just one piece of evidence**, we would need the fossil that swam from one layer to another; we would need evidence that the universe is not expanding, we need evidence that the stars appear to be far away, but they're not. We would need evidence that rock layers can somehow form in just four thousand years instead of the extraordinary number. We need evidence that somehow that you can reset the atomic clock and keep the neutrons from becoming protons. **Bring out any of those things, and you would change me immediately."**

Nye and Ham's answers demonstrate very different kinds of reasoning. Ham's reasoning is ossified and dogmatic; Nye's reasoning is flexible and open to new facts and insights. Yet it's important to note that people of Faith can also be good scientists. Below are a few examples of individuals who have apparently synthesized a working relationship between their religious beliefs and science. Flip a mental switch one way and the focus is on religion, flip the switch in the opposite direction and the focus is on science.

- **Giordano Bruno**, the Italian philosopher who proposed that "the universe has no center, and stars are suns surrounded by planets and moons. Remarkably, he thus outlined large-scale aspects of our cosmology, while Copernicus and Kepler mistakenly thought the universe is spherical, the sun is its center, unmoving, and stars are not suns surrounded by planets."[72] In 1600 Bruno was burned alive in Rome as a heretic under the purview of the Roman Inquisition.
- **Christopher Clavius**[73], a Jesuit priest, astronomer, and mathematician. Known best for his work on the Gregorian calendar, which is used around the world today. Clavius also confirmed the veracity of Galileo's celestial observations.[74] A major moon crater is named after Clavius.
- **Georges Lemaître**, Jesuit priest, theoretical physicist, mathematician, astronomer, and professor of physics at the Catholic University of Louvain. Lemaître proposed his *Big Bang* theory to explain the recession of galaxies within the framework of Albert Einstein's theory of general relativity.[75]
- **Francis Collins**, an evangelical Christian, former director of the National Institutes of Health (NIH), and a leader of the international Human Genome Project.[76] The Human Genome Project enabled researchers to *read* the complete genetic blueprint of a human being.

Too Small a God

I agree with those who opine that the God of the *Bible* is too small a god based on our current understanding of the cosmos. The Old Testament reveals a god that is easily offended, demands absolute loyalty, and resorts to violence against anyone who sees things differently. The New Testament proposes a loving God who sent his only son to sacrifice himself and to show people the way to Heaven. Both the Old and New

Testaments, focus on what is right and wrong with plenty of "thou shall" and "thou shall not" injunctions on matters both large and trivial.

The authors of the *Bible* were unaware that we live in an apparently infinite universe that is chockablock with other galaxies and worlds and held together with *dark matter* and *dark energy*.[77] The myopic view expressed in the *Bible* is not surprising given that the origins of the *Bible* span both the Bronze Age[78] and the Iron Age[79].

Embracing God as described within the framework of the *Bible* seems to me a bit like embracing what passed as medicine in Jesus' time rather than our medical knowledge today. Would you prefer an ancient physician whose toolkit includes herbs, a lance, and a limited understanding of anatomy and physiology, or a physician today who has access to advanced diagnostics, procedures, and drugs?

In the book, *The Varieties of Scientific Experience*[80], Carl Sagan makes several interesting observations about the intersection of religion and scientific inquiry, including

> "…a general problem with much of Western theology in my view is that the God portrayed is too small. It is a god of a tiny world and not a god of a galaxy, much less of a universe.
>
> Now, we can say, "Well, that's just because the right words weren't available back when the first Jewish or Christian or Islamic holy books were written." But clearly, that's not the problem; it is certainly possible in the beautiful metaphors in these books to describe something like the galaxy and the universe, and it isn't there. It is a god of one small world, a problem, I believe, that theologians have not adequately addressed.
>
> If a Creator God exists, would He or She or It or whatever the appropriate pronoun is, prefer a kind of sodden blockhead who worships while understanding nothing? Or would He prefer His votaries to admire the real universe in
> all its intricacy?"

During a television interview, Sagan was asked about his views on science and religion, and at one point Sagan asked his host,

> "Who is more humble? The scientist who looks at the universe with an open mind and accepts whatever the universe has to teach us, or somebody who says everything in this book must be considered the literal truth and never mind the fallibility of all the human beings involved?"[81]

Richard Feynman, theoretical physicist, and Nobel Prize recipient held a comparable view to Sagan of the biblical God,

> "It doesn't seem to me that this fantastically marvelous universe, this tremendous range of time and space and different kinds of animals, and all the different plants, and all these atoms with their motions and so on, all this complicated thing can merely be a stage so that God can watch human beings struggle for good and evil – which is the view that religion has. The stage is too big for the drama."[82]

As an agnostic, I would hope that a revealed god would want us to use the gifts of reason and curiosity he has given us so we can fully appreciate the universe. I would hope that if this god has any fury left, it would be for those who are willfully ignorant, who promote conspiracy theories, misinformation, and disinformation, and those who have traded their God-given gifts of reason and curiosity for the comfort of mindless submission to dogma.

Intelligent Design

Some who seek proof of God point to the concept of *intelligent design*. "The theory of intelligent design holds that certain features of the universe and of living things are best explained by an intelligent cause, not an undirected process such as natural selection."[83] Proponents of this idea state that,

> "Unlike creationism, the scientific theory of intelligent design does not claim that modern biology can identify

whether the intelligent cause detected through science is supernatural.

The theory of intelligent design, unlike creationism, is not based upon the *Bible*. Instead, it is based on observations of nature which the theory attempts to explain based on what we know about the cause-and-effect structure of the world and the patterns that generally indicate intelligent causes. Intelligent design is an inference from empirical evidence, not a deduction from religious authority."[84]

It seems to me that those who promote intelligent design maintain that a remarkably ingenious entity is involved in the creation of the temporal world, but that entity is not necessarily God. I also wonder why an "intelligent designer" would construct we humans so our own bodies can create lethal cancers? That doesn't seem like a very intelligent design choice to me.

Near-Death Experiences

Another "proof source" for God and the afterlife that's offered by some people of Faith is the *near-death* experience. In near-death experiences, an individual dies, leaves her physical body, and may be greeted by entities bathed in white light who sometimes include deceased family members. The person undergoing these experiences may be told by the spirits she meets to go back because it isn't her time to die. Occasionally miraculous recoveries are claimed by people who heed their ghostly relatives and return to the world of the living.[85, 86] For example, according to Betty Eadie's near-death experience, starting with a trip through a dark tunnel where she was met by a figure,

'It was Jesus Christ, she said. 'He hugged me and said, it's not yet your time.'

Then three women - angels - appeared and Jesus told them, show her everything she needs to know, and I was taken to the most beautiful garden I'd ever seen, like nothing I'd ever seen on Earth. 'The angels then took me around every planet and then Jesus told me I had to go back to Earth, but I didn't want to.'

Then the most beautiful man I've ever seen appeared and it was God and he told me I had to go back, and I saw my body and went back into it."[87]

To people of Faith, and those who may be sitting nearer to people of Faith than atheists, these fantastic near-death stories can be compelling and offer hope that there is eternal life after death in heaven. Of course, there's a problem determining if these are true afterlife teleporting events.

Might it be that the dying subject's mind is low on oxygen, highly stressed, and constructing a comforting illusion based on beliefs that were conveyed by their parents and community in their childhood and regularly reinforced as adults? Would Eadie describe Jesus as a middle eastern person from the time of Jesus or as a contemporary white male?[88] Why are the angels that Eadie meets women and God is a most beautiful man? And what was the point of Eadie's garden tour followed by her jaunt around our solar system? Might these features of Eadie's experience demonstrate a kind of *confirmation bias* constructed from beliefs that she's long held rather than from a supernatural event? According to Britannica, confirmation bias is

> "the tendency to process information by looking for, or interpreting, information that is consistent with one's existing beliefs. This biased approach to decision-making is largely unintentional and often results in ignoring inconsistent information. Existing beliefs can include one's expectations in a given situation and predictions about a particular outcome. People are especially likely to process information to support their own beliefs when the issue is highly important or self-relevant."[89]

Enter the *god helmet* (originally called the Koren helmet after its inventor Stanley Koren). Neuroscientist Michael Persinger[90] used a god helmet made from a modified snowmobile helmet that incorporated solenoids placed over the temporal lobes for his research. These solenoids created a weak, rotating magnetic field within the temporal lobe of the brain.

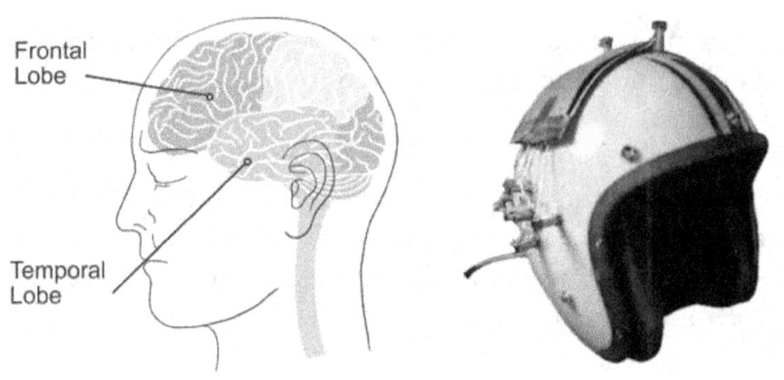

Temporal lobe (left), God Helmet[91] (right)

A journalist who experienced the god helmet reported that[92]:

- I drift almost at once into a warm bath of oblivion. Something is definitely happening.
- During the 35-minute experiment, I feel a distinct sense of being withdrawn from the envelope of my body and set adrift in an infinite existential emptiness, a deep sensation of waking slumber.
- Occasionally, I surface to an alpha state where I sort of know where I am, but not quite. This feeling is cool - like being reinserted into my body. Then there's a separation again, of body and soul, and - almost by my will - I happily allow myself to drift back to the surprisingly bearable lightness of oblivion.
- In this floating state, several ancient childhood memories are jarred loose. Suddenly, I am sitting with Scott Allen on the rug in his Colonial Street house in Charleston, South Carolina, circa 1965, singing along to "Moon River" and clearly hearing, for the first time since then, Scott's infectiously frenzied laughter.
- I reexperience the time I spent the night with Doug Appleby and the discomfort I felt at being in a house that was so punctiliously clean.
- If I had to pin down when I felt this dreamy state before - of being in the presence of something divine - it would be back then, in the euphoric, romantic hope that animated my adolescent efforts at meditation.

As authors of a paper presented at the International Conference on Modern Approach in Humanities wondered,

> "What if we could recreate a religious experience by simply flipping a switch in the brain? What if we could produce the feeling that someone or something is watching over us on demand? According to neuroscientific research conducted with The God Helmet, this may be possible.
>
> Can we artificially induce religious experiences in people? Believers never question whether or not god is real. However, it has been suggested by neuroscientists that god may in fact be a product of the human mind. Recent discoveries in neurobiology have led some scientists to believe that there may be a specific part of the brain that causes religious feelings in humans." [93, 94]

The use of magnetic fields on the brain has shown benefits, such as the Stanford Accelerated Intelligent Neuromodulation Therapy (SAINT) approach to depression.[95, 96] However, the jury is out on what, exactly the god helmet has to offer about the existence of God and the afterlife. The experiments conducted by Persinger though do seem to support the idea that near-death experiences don't necessarily prove that some supernatural event has taken place.

The Power of Prayer

It is not uncommon to have people offer their thoughts and prayers to those undergoing hardship. Frankly, **I really appreciate** it when people tell me that I am in their thoughts and prayers even though I'm not a person of Faith. I view such sentiments as heartfelt expressions of concern and support for me from others. Thanks to all such well-wishers!

For people of Faith, prayer can be a comforting practice that improves one's outlook, reduces fear and anxiety, and in doing so may help benefit one's medical outcome. Similar benefits have been attributed to meditation. At the same time, evidence-based studies intended to demonstrate the successful intervention by prayer have failed to do so.[97, 98,]

[99] Also, as a friend wryly observed, if prayer worked reliably, then certainly it would not be permitted in gambling casinos.

In the absence of objective evidence, people of Faith may turn to positive stories as *proof sources* for the power of prayer, for example,

> "We hear accounts of people in financial trouble suddenly receiving precisely the amount they need from unexpected sources…Men and women frequently pray for miracles, which do occur, including healed bodies, healed relationships, and loved ones coming to Christ."[100]

Of course, *hearing accounts of* successful interventions (*anecdotes*) is not the same as a rigorous evidence-based study. Further, it's not uncommon for miraculous claims to include only stories of success and none of the intercessory prayer failures. An example of this bias can be seen in an article about the Shrine of Our Lady of Good Help in Champion, Wisconsin.[101]

The question of prayer, especially of *intercessory* prayer that intends to change outcomes, raises curious questions for me. If God has a plan for all of us, and if God is unerring, and if my plan includes cancer, then what is the purpose of asking God to change his plan for me? Doesn't doing so suggest that the one praying doesn't accept God's wisdom and will? Why would God change his mind? Also, wouldn't a person of Faith who has led a just life look forward to entering the afterlife – why try to stay on earth when you could be in heaven?

A position expressed by Charles F. Stanley, the founder of *In Touch Ministries*, is that one does not pray to change God's plan (which is unchangeable) but rather to get into *harmony* with God. Essentially, the person praying is preparing herself so she can accept God's plan, and possibly be involved in effecting God's plan – even if the outcome is not the desired one.[102] In a similar vein, some may also recall the *Serenity Prayer*, written by the American theologian Reinhold Niebuhr which is commonly quoted as,

> "God, grant me the serenity to accept
> the things I cannot change,
> courage to change the things I can,

and wisdom to know the difference."

In a way, this acceptance of things that can't be changed and the courage to change those things which can be changed is very much in line with the Stoic philosophy that I discuss ahead in the Philosophical Perspectives section. A key difference is that the religious approach incorporates God and articles of faith whereas the philosophical approach does not. Consequently, the philosophical approach may be more meaningful and accessible to those who are not religious and to those who are questioning their Faith.

Again, I'm not trying to convert anyone or challenge their Faith in this section of the book. If prayer gives you comfort and helps you deal with your cancer diagnosis, then by all means pray!

Religious Culture

Please don't think that my observations above show my disregard for formal religions; nothing can be further from the truth. Religious institutions have expressed their Faith through spectacular art, high moral and ethical aspirations, and powerful song among other cultural features. I am still moved by religious melodies from my youth: the *Ave Maria*[103], the *Kyrie Eleison*[104], *Hark the Herald Angels Sing*[105], and other hymns and chorales.

I'm also pleasantly surprised when songs of Faith remind the faithful how the practice of their Faith can be superficial and misguided. One of my favorite artists is Gregory Porter and his song *Take Me to The Alley*.[106] This song is a challenge to ideas like "prosperity theology"[107] and a call for people of Faith to return to Jesus' message of helping those less fortunate among us. The opening verses from *Take Me to the Alley* follow,

"Well, they guild their houses
In preparation for the King
And they line the sidewalks
With every sort of shiny thing
They will be surprised
When they hear him say

Take me to the alley
Take me to the afflicted ones

97

Take me to the lonely ones
That somehow lost their ways

Let them hear me say
I am your friend
Come to my table
Rest here in my garden
You will have a pardon"

If there is a God, then I would hope that *Take Me to the Alley* is also God's favorite song, rather than another hallelujah about paying homage to a supreme being.

For me, religion offers no answers to the kinds of questions that I listed above, for example, "What did I do wrong and why am I being punished?" I view cancer as yet another one of the many probabilities that come with living in the natural world. While there are certain steps that one can take to reduce the risk of cancer (e.g., stop smoking, and avoid environmental pollutants), doing so is no guarantee that cancer will be avoided.

There is no fairness to cancer and often few means of seeking an injunction for its effects. I'm reminded of an exchange between Oberyn Martell and Tyrion Lannister, two characters in the series *Game of Thrones*, which could apply to cancer.[108]

> Martell: "And what about what I want? Justice for my sister and her children."
> Lannister: "If you want justice, you've come to the wrong place."

Philosophical Perspectives

Although religions certainly have a philosophical perspective, I view philosophy separately from religion in that it does not necessarily rely upon a supernatural entity. Further, philosophy may offer a certain formal structure and guidance, but it does not require an absolute belief in dogmatic articles of faith, congregating with others for ritual celebrations, and so forth. According to The Philosophy Foundation[109],

"Philosophy is a way of thinking about certain subjects such as ethics, thought, existence, time, meaning and value. That 'way of thinking' involves 4 Rs: responsiveness, reflection, reason, and re-evaluation. The aim is to deepen understanding. The hope is that by doing philosophy we learn to think better, to act more wisely, and thereby help to improve the quality of all our lives."

Three philosophies that influence my view of the world are Stoicism, Taoism, and the martial art of Aikido.

Stoicism

I was introduced to Stoicism a few years ago via popular books on the subject by Ryan Holiday.[110] Like many popular book authors, I feel that Holiday has created a too-simplistic representation of Greek Stoic philosophy so the topic would be appealing and accessible to the general reader – he's apparently created a successful business around his books. At the same time, I think that the core concepts discussed in Holiday's books, and in the writings of the original Stoic philosophers, are useful.

Of the various promoters of Stoicism, three men are often referred to: Epictetus,[111] Marcus Aurelius,[112] and Seneca[113]. At the heart of Stoicism is the idea that there are some things that we can control (like a healthy lifestyle) and many things that are outside of our control (like a cancer diagnosis). Therefore, we should act where we can while accepting that our best efforts may not achieve the results which we wish. Note, too, that modern cognitive behavioral therapy (CBT) has strong associations with this Stoic outlook.[114, 115]

As a side note, the term *stoic* has come to be associated with "one apparently or professedly indifferent to pleasure or pain, not affected by or showing passion or feeling."[116] This contemporary word association is misleading. The origin of the word *Stoic* provides insight into how the meaning of the term has changed over time. According to Merriam-Webster[117],

"Zeno of Citium, born in Cyprus in the 4th century B.C.E., traveled to Athens while a young man and studied with the important philosophers of the day, among them two influential Cynics.

He eventually arrived at his own philosophy and began teaching at a public hall called the Stoa Poikile. Zeno's philosophy, Stoicism, took its name from the hall where he taught, and it preached self-control, fortitude, and justice; passion was seen as the cause of all evil.

By the 14th century, English speakers had adopted the word stoic as a general term for anyone who could face adversity calmly and without excess emotion. By the 15th century, we'd also begun using it as an adjective meaning "not affected by or showing passion or feeling."

So, Stoicism began as an open-air class on philosophy and is now typically associated solely with passionless individuals. I ask that you forgo the modern meaning, so the original primary Stoic goals of self-control, fortitude, and justice are restored.

Taoism

It was during my time as an undergraduate at Scranton University that I was exposed to other religions and philosophies. I found myself leaning more toward eastern concepts, particularly Taoism and its foundational book, the *Tao Te Ching*.[118] Taoism seemed to provide me with more useful insight than the complicated and contradictory nature of Roman Catholicism.

Tao may be defined as "the unconditional and unknowable source and guiding principle of all reality as conceived by Taoists."[119] The *Tao Te Ching* is attributed to a man named Lao-Tzu[120]. Curiously, it is not clear if this person existed and was the exclusive author, or if the *Tao Te Ching* is an amalgam of thinking at the time it was written.

This question about the authorship of the *Tao Te Ching* may understandably seem a kind of unknown authorship and contradiction that I discussed about the *Bible* in the Religious Perspectives section above. However, unlike the *Bible* and other kinds of sacred scripture one is not required to believe that the true author of the *Tao Te Ching* is God and so may assess the books stanzas on their face, secular value.

Although Taoism is practiced as a religion by many, I consider its core concepts solely from the philosophical view here rather than a religious one. Taoism can be simultaneously enigmatic and insightful. Two examples from the *Tao Te Ching* follow.[121]

****

"The tao that can be told is not the eternal Tao. The
name that can be named is not the eternal Name."

****

"Therefore, the Master acts without doing anything
and teaches without saying anything.
Things arise and she lets them come;
things disappear and she lets them go.
She has but doesn't possess, acts but doesn't expect.
When her work is done, she forgets it.
That is why it lasts forever."

As the passages above show, The *Tao Te Ching* certainly doesn't offer the "thou shalt, shalt not" kind of admonishments found in the *Bible*, and some may argue that the book is no less contradictory than the *Bible* and other sacred scripture. I suggest, however, that you read the entire slim text with an open mind, pausing to reflect on the observations it makes and consider how the stanzas may apply in your life, regardless of your religious Faith.

I provide a few stanzas from the *Tao Te Ching* and quotes by Stoic philosophers and practitioners under the Wrapping it Up section.

Aikido

When I was in college, I trained for a couple of years in Tang Soo Do, a Korean style of karate that favors a variety of striking kicks. Like many other forms of self-defense, Tang Soo Do is mostly a "hard style" whereby the practitioner engages an opponent directly, blocking the opponent's strikes while working on the opponent's "inside" to land counterstrikes. For example, if an opponent throws a punch to your face, then you would block that punch, moving the opponent's arm away to

101

create an opening to land your own punch to the opponent's face or chest.

It's interesting to note that the "Do" part of Tang Soo Do "is related to the Chinese word 'tao' or 'dao,' which means 'way' or 'path.' So, Tang Soo Do, contrary to the understanding of many non-practitioners, is not a sport or a hobby. It is a way of life, a path to follow. As such, it carries with it not only techniques for striking and blocking and kicking but a philosophy for living." [122] Although such hard styles of karate are common, they are not the only approach in martial arts.

Several years ago, I took classes in Aikido, a Japanese martial arts form.[123] Unlike hard styles of karate, Aikido avoids direct and forceful contact with opponents. Instead, the Aikido practitioner works to redirect an opponent's force and thereby neutralize the threat. For example, if an opponent attempts to strike or grab you, then rather than blocking the opponent's strike to land a strike of your own, you will work to the "outside" of the opponent, redirecting the force of their attack by a throw that places the opponent in a non-threatening position.

The quote below is by Morihei Ueshiba, also known as O-Sensei and the founder of Aikido[124]. Note how his philosophy on Aikido emulates that expressed in the *Tao Te Ching*.

> "There are no contests in the Art of Peace. A true warrior
> is invincible because he or she contests with nothing."
> — *O-Sensei*

To get a sense of how Aikido differs from karate I invite you to check out a couple of stylized demonstrations, one of Tang Soo Do (https://bit.ly/3S5qteS) and the other of Aikido (https://bit.ly/3cMneJd). Note that some contend that the original form of Aikido as taught by O-Sensei is practically useless in a real street fight situation. In fact, actual combat by any martial art rarely (if ever) works as well as demonstrations like the ones above suggest, but these video examples give you a sense of how a confrontational style philosophy differs from a nonconfrontational style philosophy.

I mentioned earlier that I joined the wrestling team in my senior year of high school. High school and collegiate wrestling have features that are similar to Aikido. The sport is between two participants and no punches or kicks are allowed. Instead, the opponents *grapple* in a kind of kinetic ballet where each party is looking for an inflection point – a position and time when they can redirect their opponent's movement and energy to their advantage. A wrestler may be losing in points during competition but can still win the match by a swift and well-executed *pin* – positioning the opponent on his back for a two-second contact between both shoulders (or shoulder blades) and the mat.

From a philosophical perspective, I prefer the deescalating approach of Aikido and wrestling over the combative way of Tang Soo Do and boxing. Like my interest in Stoicism and Taoism, my basic understanding and appreciation of Aikido and my very brief time as a wrestler also influence my worldview on other topics like dealing with cancer.

***

Let's move on to the next and final main section of the book where I'll discuss how I'm currently dealing with my cancer diagnosis, treatment, and prognosis.

WRAPPING IT UP

So, with the completion of the previous section on emotional, religious, and philosophical perspectives, you now know the following three things about me:

1. I'm by nature a private and *emotionally closed* person who is reluctant to share my feelings or ask for help (but I'm trying to improve)
2. I'm an agnostic who is not convinced by the beliefs of either people of Faith or atheists. Rather, I acknowledge that either extreme view may be possible, although both are equally unlikely. I'm willing to reconsider my position if presented with reasoned, compelling evidence (not strong opinion, dogma, or *apologetics*).
3. Although I'm not an expert in Stoicism, Taoism, or Aikido I am influenced by my understanding of their core concepts. The symbiotic relationship I have in my mind with these schools of thought offers me a "go with the flow" perspective that does not rule out taking action. I act where I can while I accept that the result may not necessarily be the outcome for which I had hoped.

The three insights above ought to help explain the additional information and comments that I share below in this final section.

Summary

We've arrived at the end of this book and now I'll wrap things up and offer some closing thoughts about how I've been dealing with my cancer therapy and prognosis. Let's first start with a summary of the information covered in the book up to this point.

- Cancer is a disease in which some of the body's cells grow uncontrollably and spread to other parts of the body.
- There is no single cause of cancer. Scientists believe that it is the interaction of many factors together that produces cancer. The

factors involved may be genetic, environmental, or constitutional characteristics of the individual.

- Pancreatic cancer is cancer that originates in the pancreas. If pancreatic cancer spreads or grows to other organs like the liver (metastasizes), then it is also referred to as pancreatic rather than liver cancer.

- Due to the normally late detection and effectiveness of current pancreatic cancer therapies, the outlook is frankly bleak.

- Survival rates can give you an idea of what percentage of people with the same type and stage of cancer are still alive for a certain amount of time, but survival rates can't tell you how long you will live; they can't predict what will happen in any particular person's case.

- There are common procedures that cancer patients will undergo, including blood workup, CT and MRI scans, endoscopy procedures, and placement of an access port for infusions.

- Patient journeys include first signs of trouble, diagnosis, a program of therapy, side effects from the therapy, and unexpected bumps along the way.

- Getting a cancer diagnosis raises emotional, religious, and philosophical issues, especially regarding our mortality. These issues affect not only the cancer patient but the patient's family and friends.

- Each cancer patient is different from the nature of their cancer and their response to therapy to the way they view the world and deal with their diagnosis and prognosis.

- I recognize that your experiences aren't the same as mine, and I don't presume that you will agree with my perspective or that my approach is "right" for you. Perhaps, however, some of what I offer might be of some practical use to you and yours.

Dealing with Cancer

One of the main things that others want to know from a cancer patient is how they are dealing with their disease. By *dealing with*, I mean how the patient is managing the emotional and physical ups and downs, especially when faced with the typically poor prognosis of pancreatic cancer. This may not be a question that is directly asked of you but rather implied by questions like "How are you holding up?" or statements like "I can't imagine how difficult this is for you."

As I regularly remind the reader throughout this book, every cancer patient is different and so is their personal journey. How one cancer patient may be dealing with their disease very likely isn't the same way that other cancer patients are dealing with their disease.

In the Emotional, Religious, and Philosophical Perspectives section of this book, I shared with you my own experiences and thoughts as a way to set a foundation for how I'm dealing with my disease. The core elements of my approach include acknowledging that while I can (and should) act where I'm able, there are many things outside of my control. I can certainly guess about the future and fret over what may happen, or I can keep my focus on today and what's actually happening around me.

Rather than offering you some kind of simple but dubious 10-step plan, allow me to walk you through several additional observations and thoughts below. Consider this walkabout a kind of informal chat between us that's intended to get you thinking about your own journey, how you are dealing (or not dealing) with your disease now, and how you might modify your current mindset to improve your outlook.

Keep in mind, too, an observation that Steven Merlin regularly makes – cancer is *treatable*. This isn't to suggest that current treatments are curative (although they sometimes are), rather that there are a variety of therapeutic options available today and you certainly can engage with those therapies instead of throwing up your arms in surrender to your disease.

Postponing the Inevitable

It may surprise you to learn that "There are many theories about the mechanisms of age-related changes, and they are mutually exclusive, no one theory is sufficiently able to explain the process of aging, and they often contradict one another."[125] In other words, we know that our bodies grow old and die (a process known as *senescence*[126]) but we don't really understand why this is the case.

The theories try to describe the cause and nature of aging, exploring both the biological and psychological realms. At the end of the day, and regardless of the reasons for why we age, the process of aging may be represented by my simple diagram below.

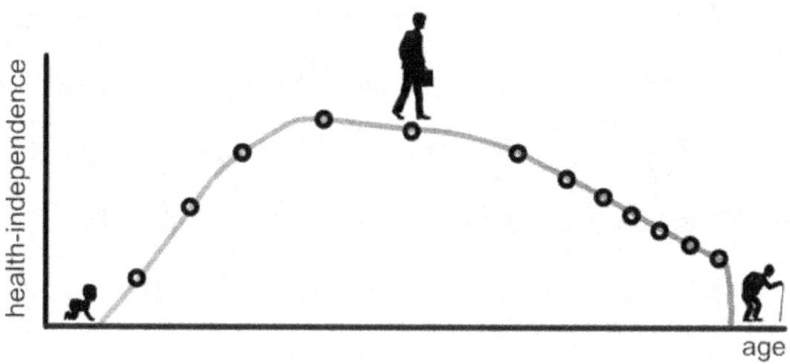

In the diagram above, the x-axis is the age of an individual, ranging from birth on the left to death on the right. The y-axis is what I refer to as *health-independence*, a combination of the physical and mental health of an individual and the independence of the individual based on their health. Let's start at the left side of the diagram with the crawling baby and move to the right side of the diagram with the senior icon for an individual whom we'll call Sam.

Assuming a normal birth, Sam starts out life in good health but needs constant care. The healthy infant Sam left to his own devices would not last long in the world, consequently, his health-independence is low. As Sam ages through puberty and enters his 20s, he encounters occasional health issues like the flu or a broken bone (indicated by the black circles along the health-independence line). Sam also becomes more independent in the sense that he can make health decisions himself, including a healthy diet and exercise. Sam's health-independence peaks as he heads toward middle age, and then starts to decline as more health issues arise such as high blood pressure and diabetes which start to reduce his health-independence.

Aging further into his senior years, Sam encounters increasingly more frequent and serious health issues such as heart, kidney, and joint disease that further diminish his health-independence. In the latter part of Sam's senior years' other doors open to more serious diseases like cancer, neurological disorders, and dementia. The higher frequency of these diseases is indicated in the diagram by the shorter distance between black dots on the health-independence line). The *compression of morbidity theory*[127] suggests that if chronic illnesses can be pushed forward in Sam's life, then he may have a longer lifespan. At some point, however, Sam's body can no longer compensate for the effects of his diseases, and Sam dies.

Of course, unforeseen events like accidents and other medical issues can occur at any time throughout anyone's life. You may have your own stories about an otherwise healthy friend or family member who had a lethal fall in the shower or dropped dead of a sudden cardiac arrest while shoveling snow.

If there were a cure for cancer tomorrow and all we cancer patients returned to our original, pre-cancerous path, then we would still be vulnerable to other diseases and accidents – just like everyone else. There simply isn't any way of avoiding our death. If there is a "silver lining" in an event that takes one's life sooner than expected, then perhaps it is that a multitude of other unpleasant diseases like Alzheimer's and ALS are also avoided.

I'm confident that in the years ahead, effective therapies for cancers and many more diseases will appear. In the long game, however, Death picks the time and place and always wins. We can eat healthily and exercise, or we can abuse our bodies. We can die while shoveling snow or be one of the few people who are successfully resuscitated from a sudden cardiac arrest to live another day.[128] However, even with our best efforts and the skilled intervention by health care professionals, we are all simply postponing the inevitable. You can fight this fact or get used to it so it doesn't consume your focus and cause you to miss the good things that you can experience daily.

On Life and Death

And I am not frightened of dying
Any time will do, I don't mind
Why should I be frightened of dying?
There's no reason for it, you've gotta go sometime
– *The Great Gig in the Sky*, Pink Floyd

I don't disagree with the sentiment of the lyrics above; dying is just part of life and we've all got to go sometime. However, we tend to go about our daily business as if our days will continue forever. We agonize over work demands and managing family issues well into the future, although all around us we see our fellow humans making their departures. Perhaps we don't dwell on our mortality because we fear it and we keep our dread at bay by avoiding the topic all together. We may feel that by acknowledging our mortality we would be "giving up" – why go on if the is no way to avoid our certain end?

I don't believe that accepting one's mortality is "giving up." Rather, acceptance can enable you to focus on the here and now, to appreciate the good things that happen on your good days however many days remain for you. The following joke was shared with me by an old friend and is a good reminder of how we miss the obvious when our attention is distracted:

Tell Me What You See

Sherlock Holmes and Dr. Watson were camping. After dinner and a bottle of wine, they lay down for the night, and go to sleep. Later, Holmes awakes and nudges his faithful friend.

"Watson, look up at the sky and tell me what you see."

Watson replies, "I see millions of stars."

"What does that tell you?"

Watson ponders the question for a minute and replies.,

"Astronomically, it tells me that there are millions of galaxies and potentially billions of planets."

"Astrologically, I observe that Saturn is in Leo."

"Horologically, I deduce that the time is approximately a quarter past three."

"Theologically, I can see that God is all-powerful and that we are small and insignificant."

"Meteorologically, I suspect that we will have a beautiful day tomorrow."

"What does it tell you, Holmes?" Watson asked.

Holmes replies, "Watson, you idiot. Someone has stolen our tent!"

Riding the Rollercoasters

When I was a kid, our family was vacationing at the Maryland shore, taking in the summer boardwalk of food vendors, games of skill, and rides. One of the popular rides was the *Wild Mouse* rollercoaster and people seemed to be having fun, so I asked to go on the ride, too. I handed a soda that I was drinking to my mother, got in line, and boarded the rollercoaster.

Wild Mouse had narrow cars that made their way along a narrow track. After the initial climb, the cars noisily snake their way through a series of hairpin curves. The design of the ride creates the illusion that the cars may fall sideways off the track or miss a tight turn and go straight over the edge. These hairpin turns are followed by a series of drops and banked turns that return the rider to the start point.[129]

I was so shaken by the experience that when I got off the ride, I had to use both hands to control the soda that my mother returned to me. I decided at once to never go on a rollercoaster again, and my promise lasted until I was about forty years old.

Around the time that I turned forty, I was recovering from a series of setbacks: a job loss, a divorce, selling a house in central New Jersey, and relocating to a one-bedroom garden apartment in north New Jersey near the New York state border. During this time, I decided to try a variety of activities that I hadn't experienced on my way to my middle age. Skiing (downhill, cross-country, telemark), hiking, screenwriting, and so forth. As I sampled these various activities, Diane was playing along by arranging surprise adventures into New York City and attractions around New Jersey. One of her adventures was to Six Flags Great Adventure.

Walking around the park we spied *Batman*, a new tortuous rollercoaster ride at the time. The ride seats were suspended from a track above the riders, so riders' legs dangled and swung freely below. A first steep drop went directly into a 360-degree loop that led into a 360-degree corkscrew followed by more dips and rises, all of which created an illusion of flying with reckless abandon. *Batman* was to *Wild Mouse* what several shots-and-a-beer is to a weak near-beer.

Of course, my natural inclination was to just walk by this monstrosity, but in the spirit of trying new things, Diane and I got into a long line for the ride. There were actually two lines: one for those who wanted to brave the front seats for an unobstructed view, and another faster line that would lead to seats in the middle and back. We got into the front seat line.

The ride was everything that its design promised. Although I had told myself for decades that I would never take another rollercoaster ride, I embraced the experience, hands grasping the harness and yelling all the way. After the ride finished, I realized that what I had feared and avoided for so many years wasn't what I imagined it would be. Diane and I got back into the front seat line again.

"Okay, Bob," you may be asking, "What do rollercoasters have to do with cancer?" Well, try the following analogy on for size.

Think about a cancer diagnosis like a park full of rides. Instead of rollercoasters, cancer rides include therapies, their side effects, various procedures, and emotional blows. The fact that you are in this cancer park means that you've been diagnosed with cancer – you didn't choose to be at the park but here you are. You have, however, decided to fight your cancer by choosing to ride the rollercoaster of therapies, procedures, and emotional swings.

You've likely gotten an x-ray in the past even if only at the dentist, but other procedures you'll encounter may be new, alarming, and downright scary for you. In this fearful state of mind, you are like the kid who just shakily climbed out of the *Wild Mouse*.

As time goes on and you become familiar with the rollercoasters of therapies, procedures, and emotions you become more like the adult who rides in the front seats of *Batman*. Of course, you'd rather not be in the park or ride the rollercoasters, however, you somehow handle the experience better through repetition and gain important insights into your ability to deal with adversity.

> When those days occur where you are the shaky kid on the *Wild Mouse* don't beat yourself up. Tomorrow – or the next day, you'll take on the *Batman* again.

Selected Quotes

I'm generally not a fan of quotes. They are often too simplistic to be useful, especially when they are taken out of context and embraced as incontrovertible truths – particularly when they involve life and death issues. For the purposes of this section of the book, however, I hope that the few quotes and comments offered below might be thought-provoking and helpful to you. These quotes come from a variety of sources, including Stoic philosophers, the *Tao Te Ching*, scriptwriters, the CEO of an infant bereavement non-profit, and other cancer patients.

Stoic Philosophers

- The final hour when we cease to exist does not itself bring death; it merely of itself completes the death process. We reach death at that moment, but we have been a long time on the way. (Seneca)

- Don't behave as if you are destined to live forever. Death hangs over you. While you live, while it is in your power, be good. Now. (Marcus Aurelius)

- I cannot escape death, but at least I can escape the fear of it. (Epictetus)

- What is death? A scary mask. Take it off – see, it doesn't bite. Eventually, body and soul will have to separate, just as they existed separately before we were born. So why be upset if it happens now? If it isn't now, it's later. (Epictetus)

- What upsets people is not things themselves but their judgments about the things. For example, death is nothing dreadful, but instead, the judgment about death is what is dreadful. So, when we are thwarted or upset or distressed, let us never blame someone else but rather ourselves, that is, our own judgments. (Epictetus)

- Accept death in a cheerful spirit, as nothing but the dissolution of the elements from which each living thing is composed. If it doesn't hurt the individual elements to change continually into one another, why are people afraid of all of them changing and separating? It's a natural thing. And nothing natural is evil. (Marcus Aurelius)

The Tao Te Ching

- Immersed in the wonder of the Tao, you can deal with whatever life brings you, and when death comes, you are ready.

- The Master gives himself up to whatever the moment brings. He knows that he is going to die, and he has nothing left to hold on to: no illusions in his mind, no resistance in his body. He doesn't think about his actions; they flow from the core of his being. He holds nothing back from life; therefore, he is ready for death, as a man is ready for sleep after a good day's work.

- If you realize that all things change, there is nothing you will try to hold on to. If you aren't afraid of dying, there is nothing you can't achieve. Trying to control the future is like trying to take the master carpenter's place. When you handle the master carpenter's tools, chances are that you'll cut your hand.

Good Will Hunting

Dealing with the challenges of pancreatic cancer can cause you to feel weak and powerless. A little *snarky* attitude toward your cancer may be a good way to vent your frustrations.

In the movie, *Good Will Hunting*[130], there is a scene between Will and his therapist, Sean. Will relates how his father would use corporal punishment including making Will and his brother collect sticks from a local park. Will's father would put a belt, a stick that his sons provided, and a wrench onto the kitchen table and tell his children to choose their punishment.

Sean assumes that Will would have selected the belt – perhaps the least brutal form of punishment offered, but Will tells Sean he chose the wrench. "The wrench, why?" Sean asks. "Cause fuck him, that's why," Will replies.

Cancer and chemotherapy don't offer the cancer patient the opportunity to choose the kind of physical punishment that the disease and treatments will deliver. If they did, then patients would certainly choose the metaphorical *belt* over the *wrench*. Adopting a snarky attitude toward whatever cancer and chemotherapy throws your way can be extraordinarily difficult. Telling the disease "Fuck you," however, may be a small but empowering gesture that you can take. Give it a try!

Jackie

The dialog below is from the 2016 movie, Jackie[131]. In the scene, Jackie Kennedy is sharing with her priest how difficult it is for her to continue after the assassination of her husband, President John F. Kennedy. Although the priest in the film does not represent an actual priest, the dialog may reflect exchanges that Jackie had with the Jesuit priest Rev. Richard McSorley[132, 133]. Although I'm not a person of Faith, being raised as a Catholic (and trained by Jesuits along the way), this passage "rings true" to me.

> "There comes a time in man's search for meaning, when one realizes – there are no answers. When you come to that horrible, unavoidable realization – you accept it. Or you kill yourself. Or you simply stop searching.
>
> I have lived a blessed life. And yet every night when I climb into bed, turn off the lights, and stare into the dark,

I wonder...is this all there is? Every soul on this planet does.

And then, when morning comes, we all wake up and make a pot of coffee. Because we do. You did this morning, and you will again tomorrow. God, in his infinite wisdom, has made sure....it is just enough for us."

Zoe Clark-Coates

Clark-Coates co-founded the charity *The Mariposa Trust* (widely known by the name of its primary division *sayinggoodbye.org*) with her husband Andy.[134] Although the non-profit mission is about bereavement for those who lose a baby, the quote below has a Stoic perspective that is similar to the Jackie dialog above. I feel Clark-Coates' perspective below also applies to cancer patients when they find themselves in a low spot.

"You made it another day, even though yesterday you did
not feel you could survive another hour.
Right now, you may laugh if I called you a warrior, but
that is what you are.
You are moving forward little by little; even though you
do not want to.
When your heart is telling you to just curl into a ball and
never move again, you say no, and you still get dressed
and face each day."

Cancer Patients' Perspectives

Listening to the views of other cancer patients about how they are dealing with their disease may provide useful insights that you hadn't considered. You may also find that stories similar to yours are comforting because you are reminded that others share your experience, challenges, and fears.

Rachel May

The following is a public post made on LinkedIn by Rachel Mae, who identified herself at the time as a sales professional who celebrated her one year of being cancer free[135]. I feel that Rachel has captured the essence of what many people with cancer, including me, come to know.

"I hate the term "live like you are dying." I know what it feels like to be dying. Trust me, it's not about skydiving and bucket lists. Living like you're dying looks a lot more like fighting for one more day to live.

For one more day to memorize your child's face, touch your partner's skin, lay in cold grass, smell the season, hear the wind rustle through the trees.

When you are dying, you don't seek out the most extraordinary day before you go. You hold on to one more ordinary day. Just like the one you probably woke up to today.

When you are dying, you realize that the most beautiful gifts of living are in the in between. They happen every day there is breath in your lungs.

We miss them when we think our life has to be bigger. We have to see more, do more, have more to really live our best life. We sleepwalk through the living.

When you're dying, you realize the ordinary every day is in fact extraordinary. That's when you start living.

Don't live like you're dying. Live like you're living. Because today you are. This ordinary day is a miracle.

Live.""

116

DJ Stewart

DJ Stewart is a skateboarder and business owner who was diagnosed with glioblastoma, an aggressive type of cancer that begins in the brain. Stewart was profiled in the short video; *Live Like You're Dying*.[136] The following comments are excerpts from that video.

> "There are no *good* tumors, but glioblastoma is the one that's really bad and mine is a grade four. Standard prognosis, thirteen to eighteen months.
>
> You don't want to believe it. I truly just lived in it, it's like well I'm sick, guess that's my life now. And that's probably what my life would be, but it's not.
>
> So how do you fight? The biggest thing I can do to fight is just live my life, man. I try to live the absolute most normal life that I can. I just happen to be "sick."
>
> There's no fucking way that I've gotten this far to just let some dumbass cell in my brain take it away. That's bullshit."

Diane Ronnau

The late Diane Ronnau was a producer at CBS for various programs, including *48 Hours, CBS Sunday Morning,* and *CBS Evening News.* She passed in July of 2022 after a sixteen-year battle with pancreatic cancer.[137] Following are excerpts from a 2007 interview with Ronnau[138].

> "The truth is you sometimes just do things because you have to do them. I'm sick but I also have responsibilities; I have a family, I have work.
>
> As much as I was extremely worried about being sick, I also wanted to participate in the rest of my life that I'm very attached to.

Things have to be compartmentalized, you have to remember that it's time to work and then it's time to be a patient – to keep those things separate.

How do you make phone calls and set up interviews when all the time you're thinking 'I have cancer and could die'? The answer is really that it's better to persevere through those things than it is to become lost in being a cancer victim.

I'd much rather be cooking dinner, cleaning my house, taking care of my family, and going to work than being sick. If there's a distraction which is what all these things really become – things to keep you from thinking about that you're sick, they're very welcome.

You can either be identified by your illness or you can be identified by something else. I chose to not be identified by cancer."

***

You might want to pause for a moment and consider if and how any of the quotes above might help you deal better with your situation. Will you live like you're dying or live like you're living? Will you choose to be identified by your cancer or as someone who perseveres by embracing normal daily activities like family and work? Will you curl into a ball and never move again or get dressed and face each day?

A Final Word (for now)

Over my decades-long career, I created a lot of plans, projection models, financial forecasts, and other kinds of *predictions*. These exercises required that I first gather up a lot of disparate but related information such as third-party market reports, historical sales figures, customer insights, opinions of sales personnel, comments made by influencers, and so forth. I would then synthesize this pile of information into a narrative that was intended to explain with enough detail, but without overwhelming the reader, why what I thought might happen in the weeks, months and years ahead was well reasoned and ought to be pursued.

Make no doubt about it, although my presentations included tables of facts and numbers with pretty charts, it was really a work of fiction – as are all such efforts. Why create such fiction? Because some attempt to look into the future and plan is essential in any effort, so everyone involved knows what path will be taken, why the path was selected, and their role in the journey. This marriage of prediction and planning is useful not only in business but also in our personal lives.

It's easy, however, to start to believe that your fabrications about the future will absolutely come true. I've been guilty of this self-delusion myself only to find that I got things wrong and had to make changes to the narrative. It's for this reason that I've long advised others to remember a caution from statistician George Box[139],

> "…all models are wrong, but some are useful. However, the approximate nature of the model must always be borne in mind."

Put another way, to avoid the trap of self-delusion we must keep challenging our assumptions and refine our outlook as new information and understanding are obtained. We must try to confirm that our models and predictions truthfully reflect what's happening in the real world.

As I write these closing comments, I'm just past the halfway mark of my therapy – and coincidentally, also celebrated my birthday at the end of July. If I were asked to create a narrative of my future like the ones I've created in the past (based on the survival rates discussed under

Pancreatic Cancer by the Numbers), then I would predict that my cancer will probably kill me sooner than later, possibly before my next birthday. As I explained under the *Pancreatic Cancer by the Numbers* section, however, my first prediction is subject to the quirks of how individual patients respond to their therapy. Further, any estimate of survivability is confounded by Box's warning about the *wrongness* of useful models. The fact is that all sorts of things can and do confound even the most thoughtful and earnest predictions by modern-day oracles.

Although my cancer likely can't be *cured* today it's possible that I may be one of those patients like Robert Duran[140] who respond well to therapy and beat the typical survival estimate. I may find a clinical trial that produces remarkable results like those experienced by Steven Merlin,[141] Kathy Wilkes,[142] or Lynne Holcomb[143]. It's also possible that a new and more effective therapy currently under development will be approved by FDA and be available to all pancreatic cancer patients.

There simply isn't any way of knowing with certainty what lies ahead. This observation is not intended to create false hope, but simply to acknowledge that I don't have an expiration date stamped on my forehead, and I'd bet that you don't have one either.

Things change, and so my current thinking and outlook as expressed in this book may change, too, depending on how my therapy pans out. As time goes on, will I be worn down by the challenges of my disease, decide that I've had enough, and forego further treatment? Will I have a religious epiphany and return to the Catholic faith or embrace one of the many other formal religions? Those are issues that I'll have to deal with when it's time to cross those bridges.

In the meantime, my plan is to continue to take one day at a time and to focus on the here and now. As long as the quality of my life is good, I'll continue to do those things that give me a challenge and pleasure. My next project, for example, is to try my hand at woodworking and create some hand-crafted Christmas gifts for my family.

Finally, I'll leave you with another quote as a bookend to the one by Marcus Aurelius that I included in the Dedication section of this book. The quote below by novelist Jack London "is generally known as London's Credo. He is known to have said these words, just two months before his death, to a group of friends with whom he was discussing life and living."[144]

The proper function of man is to live, not to exist.
I shall not waste my days in trying to prolong them.
I shall use my time."
— Jack London, American novelist

****

If you haven't already read A Peek Through the Keyhole under the Appendices section, then I invite you to learn a bit more about Diane, our canine companions, and me.

I am open to sharing my further experiences and thoughts that arise in the weeks and months ahead as my time and health permit. I'm also interested to learn about any errors or omissions in this book so I can make corrections accordingly. I can be reached via my LinkedIn page, https://www.linkedin.com/in/robertkoshinskie

Depending on how my therapy goes, and my physical and mental abilities, I intend to revise this book sometime in the future. In the meantime, I invite you to follow me at https://www.caringbridge.org/visit/robertkoshinskie

⌒

APPENDICES

Amenities List

Creating a comfortable and comforting environment during your therapy can help deflect some of the blows of the disease and treatment.

As I explained in Family and Friends, our house was reorganized to accommodate our son staying with us. Diane uses the master bedroom, our son a guest bedroom that also serves as his office, and I use another bedroom where my laptop is set up on a small desk. This reorganization was primarily because I had to distance myself from others until the infusions were released from my body. Everyone has their own space with little interference from each other's daily activities.

Likewise, you can reorganize your living space as best meets your needs. You can also assemble items you already have and add to them with small purchases to create "kits" for hospital and home use. The table below includes suggestions for items that may offer you comfort and pleasurable distractions.

Oven mitts, useful if you are experiencing sharp pain when touching cold items	A coffee mug with an inspiring or funny slogan	Comfortable clothes and no-tie shoes (e.g., clogs, loafers)
Books, magazines, and newspapers	Pictures and photographs with special meaning to you	Air fresheners that are agreeable to you
A head cap that is UV protective with air vents	Food/beverage treats that you find appealing	Streaming music, podcasts, and movies
Puzzles, cards, and other distracting pastimes, the hospital	Wet wipes: helpful to maintain hygiene	If you have experienced diarrhea, then you might want to wear

will likely provide a television		disposable underwear to your therapy like Depend® or Tranquility® and bring an extra pair if you fear you'll experience urgent diarrhea
Suspenders: helpful for weight loss	Rachet belt: helpful for weight loss, these belts don't use holes in fixed locations – see https://amzn.to/3ocRDmj	A comfortable chair or sofa with a soft "doughnut cushion" for hard chairs and a lightweight blanket
An insulated lunch bag for hospital infusion sessions	A standard thermos for coffee and other beverages, and a wide-mouth thermos for soups and other hot foods for hospital infusion sessions	Paper, pen, and envelope to hand write a letter to family, an old friend, and others to let them know how you are doing and how much you appreciate their support

If you find that your chemotherapy significantly limits your physical abilities such as the distance you can safely walk, then you ought to look into getting a Disability Placard – those blue cards with a white wheelchair that hangs from an automobile rearview mirror. You can obtain information online on how to obtain a placard, including a form that your physician will need to provide (see the Suggested Resources section for how it's done in North Carolina).

Planning Documents

I daresay that many, if not most people associate documents like wills, advanced care directives, and power of attorney with the elderly and the infirmed. In our years into middle age, we are busy with our families, jobs, and day-to-day challenges. Why spend time and energy on documents that apply to events that won't occur for many, many years in the future?

Of course, the fact is that none of us know the date when we will "shuffle off this mortal coil."[145] Creating and maintaining key documents even starting in one's twenties serves several purposes. For one, should something happen to you unexpectedly, then your wishes are clearly and formally articulated. For another, the process of thinking through answers that these planning documents raise ought to help remind you of your mortality and responsibilities to others in your life. Leaving unfinished business to your family just adds to the burden that they bear when you pass.

The following is a brief overview of two key documents, the Living Will and the Advanced Care Directive. There is some overlap in what these documents address, and more information can be found elsewhere, including on the Mayo Clinic website[146], the National Institute on Aging[147], and the Family Care Alliance[148].

> **Note** that while these planning documents can be created via online services, I recommend that you have an attorney review such documents to ensure that they properly articulate your wishes and are compliant with requirements in your state.

Living Will

"A living will is a written, legal document that spells out medical treatments you would and would not want to be used to keep you alive, as well as your preferences for other medical decisions, such as pain management or organ donation."[149] Included in this document are your wishes regarding end-of-life care decisions such as:

- cardiopulmonary resuscitation (CPR) and the use of a defibrillator to restart your heart

- mechanical ventilation if you are unable to breathe
- feeding you nutrients and fluids intravenously or via a tube in the stomach
- dialysis when your kidneys no longer function
- use of antibiotics and antiviral medications to treat infections
- comfort care (palliative care) to keep you comfortable and manage pain

Note that do not resuscitate (DNR) and do not intubate (DNI) orders can be included in your living will or be written separately into your medical records so the hospital where you are being treated has ready access.

The Advance Health Care Directive (ADHC)

An ADHC "allows you to appoint someone (health care agent, attorney-in-fact, proxy, or surrogate) to make a decision for you if you cannot speak for yourself. It is also called the Durable Power of Attorney (POA) for Health Care, Natural Death Act, Directive to Physicians, or a Living Will. (The living will is slightly different; check on what is recognized in your state.) Every state recognizes the ADHC, but states have their own forms, as laws vary from state to state."[150] The ADHC enables a third party to work on your behalf, including but not limited to:

- Make decisions regarding any treatment, not just life-sustaining treatment
- Start helping you before you are incapacitated if you specify this is what you want
- Select or discharge care providers and institutions
- Accept or refuse specific treatments
- Withdraw or withhold life-sustaining treatment
- Allow, restrict, or forbid autopsy, unless required by law
- Direct the disposition of remains and make funeral or memorial plans

Note that your assigned POA "cannot access your medical records as long as you are competent to make your own health care decisions. AHCD is not a release of information. The Health Insurance Portability and Accountability Act (HIPAA) protect your privacy unless you sign a release of information with the treating physician. However, medical systems sometimes recognize the AHCD as a de facto release of information."

Departure Plan Example

See also <u>My Departure Plan and Housecleaning</u> section.

- ☐ Speak with your financial planner to discuss how your prognosis may affect your short- and long-term assumptions and plan
- ☐ Organize any information related to your financial plan, taxes, and other monetary topics
- ☐ Copy and organize information onto a thumb drive (e.g., wills and advance health care directive)
- ☐ Ensure that all auto-renewal links are switched to a banking account that your spouse or significant other can access
- ☐ Change information for autopay and deposit links to a banking account that your spouse or significant other can access (e.g., checking account, Venmo account, Zoom)
- ☐ Clean up and organize your personal and business email (e.g., Gmail offers categories you can set and assign individual emails)
- ☐ Clean up and organize your Microsoft and Google cloud drives
- ☐ Provide your spouse or significant other with the password for your passwords vault (see also <u>Password Managers</u> under Appendices)
- ☐ Create a family, friends, and associates email list so your spouse or significant other can send out notices as needed
- ☐ Explore hospice care (external vs. home) under Medicare A
- ☐ Conclude funeral arrangements to align with your will
- ☐ Beneficiary collects your life insurance policy
- ☐ Designated Power of Attorney distributes certain personal effects to select individuals that may not be itemized in your will (consider updating your will with these specific assignments if they have high value and/or sentimental value to multiple recipients)
- ☐ Stop inappropriate automatic payments (e.g., Medicare, auto insurance)
- ☐ Have your spouse maintain and monitor your cell phone activity for a year to ensure that your spouse receives any dual authentication requests from sites like banking, Venmo, etc.

Drug Reference

During therapy, you will receive both chemotherapy drugs and other drugs that are used to help mitigate side effects of the chemotherapy like nausea, constipation, and pain. Below I offer a quick review of some of the drugs that I've used during my therapy. The information offered was obtained from several sources like NIH National Library of Medicine Medline Plus and the American Cancer Society. Note that your therapy may or may not include the drugs listed and your side effects may or may not include those itemized below.

> The simple descriptions in this section **are not intended as medical advice**. The side effects excerpts below do not include all possible side effects included from the referenced source.
>
> **Never** rely on "Dr. Google." **Always** discuss your therapy with your health care team who can explain in detail the purpose of the different drugs, the potential side effects, and steps you can take to reduce the side effects of your therapies.

Chemotherapy Drugs

Oxaliplatin

According to MedlinePlus[151],

- Oxaliplatin is used with other medications to treat advanced colon or rectal cancer (cancer that begins in the large intestine).
- Oxaliplatin is also used with other medications to prevent colon cancer from spreading in people who have had surgery to remove the tumor.
- Oxaliplatin is in a class of medications called platinum-containing antineoplastic agents. It works by killing cancer cells.
- Oxaliplatin comes as a solution (liquid) to be injected into a vein. Oxaliplatin is administered by a doctor or nurse. It is usually given once every fourteen days.

- Oxaliplatin may cause side effects. Tell your doctor if any of these symptoms are severe or do not go away:

numbness, burning or tingling in the fingers, toes, hands, feet, mouth, or throat	pain in the hands or feet
increased sensitivity, especially to cold	decreased sense of touch
nausea	vomiting
diarrhea	constipation

Some side effects can be serious. If you experience any of these symptoms, contact your health care team at once:

stumbling or loss of balance when walking	difficulty with everyday activities such as writing or fastening buttons
difficulty speaking	strange feeling in the tongue
tightening of the jaw	chest pain or pressure
cough	shortness of breath

Irinotecan

According to MedlinePlus[152],

- Irinotecan is used alone or in combination with other medications to treat colon or rectal cancer (cancer that begins in the large intestine).
- Irinotecan is in a class of antineoplastic medications called topoisomerase I inhibitors. It works by stopping the growth of cancer cells.
- Irinotecan comes as a liquid to be given over 90 minutes intravenously (into a vein) by a doctor or nurse. It is usually given not more often than once a week, according to a schedule that alternates one or more weeks when you receive irinotecan with one or more weeks when you do not receive the medication. Your doctor will choose the schedule that will work best for you.

- Your doctor may need to delay your treatment and adjust your dose if you experience certain side effects. Be sure to tell your doctor how you are feeling during your treatment with irinotecan.
- Your doctor may give you medication to prevent nausea and vomiting before you receive each dose of irinotecan. Your doctor may also give you other medication(s) to prevent or treat other side effects.

Irinotecan may cause side effects. Tell your doctor if any of these symptoms are severe or do not go away:

Nausea, vomiting	pain, especially back pain
constipation	swelling and sores in the mouth
heartburn	loss of appetite
weight loss	hair loss
weakness	sleepiness

Some side effects can be serious. If you experience any of these symptoms, contact your health care team at once:

chest pain	yellowing of the skin or eyes
swollen stomach	unexpected or unusual weight gain
swelling of the arms, hands, feet, ankles, or lower legs	Rash, hives, itching, difficulty breathing or swallowing

Fluorouracil (5FU)

According to Cancer Research UK[153],

- Fluorouracil is also known as FU or 5FU and is one of the most commonly used drugs to treat cancer. It is most often used in combination with other cancer drugs to treat many types of cancer, including:

breast cancer	head and neck cancers
anal cancer	stomach cancer

| colon cancer | some skin cancers (as a cream) |

- Fluorouracil is part of a group of chemotherapy drugs known as anti-metabolites.
- Anti-metabolites are similar to normal body molecules, but they have a slightly different structure.
- These differences mean that anti metabolites stop cancer cells from working properly. They stop the cells from making and repairing DNA.
- Cancer cells need to make and repair DNA so that they can grow and multiply.
- You usually have fluorouracil as part of a course of several cycles of treatment. You generally have up to 6 cycles of treatment. Each cycle lasts 2, 3, or 4 weeks.
- You have continuous treatment through a small portable pump. The nurse attaches it to your central line. This means you can go home with it. You go back to the hospital regularly for the nurse to change your pump (or via homecare nursing) and to see how you're doing.

Common side effects that happen in more than 10 in 100 people (more than 10%). You might have one or more of them. They include:

Increased risk of getting an infection	Looking pale and breathlessness
Increased risk of bleeding and bruising	Feeling or being sick, diarrhea
Stiff, painful joints	Difficulty breathing.
Sore inflamed mouth and throat	Heart problems, swollen ankles
Hair loss	Loss of appetite
Soreness, redness, and peeling of palms and soles (hand-foot syndrome	Tiredness and feeling weak

Toxicity of Chemotherapy

Current chemotherapy is delivered *systemically*, meaning that it affects the patient's entire body rather than one specific organ. As explained above, chemotherapy may be infused directly into the patient's bloodstream via an infusion access port. Circulating through the patient's body the chemotherapy reaches every cell and organ from the patient's head to toe.

Chemotherapy drugs are intended to interfere with the ability of cells to multiply – which is what cancer cells are actively doing. Like "carpet bombing" chemotherapy drops its lethal payload over a large area, intending to devastate the enemy that is cancer but also creating unwanted collateral damage to healthy cells. This unintended harm occurs because some organs in the body are also multiplying for normal repair. These organs include hair follicles, bone marrow, the lining of the mouth, and the intestines. The effect of chemotherapy drugs on these normal organs is what contributes to hair loss, low white blood cell counts, mouth sores, and gastrointestinal issues.

Research continues exploring so-called *targeted therapies* that are intended to seek out just the cancer cells and thereby avoid normal cells in the body. In this respect, targeted therapies are more like guided missiles that strike an intended objective and lower the risk of collateral damage. These targeted therapies include some interesting work with mRNA technology like that used to create effective COVID-19 vaccinations. Evolving therapies are outside the scope of this book, and you can learn more on the National Cancer Institute website[154, 155] and elsewhere.[156]

According to the American Cancer Society (ACS)[157], "Chemotherapy drugs are considered to be hazardous to people who handle them or come into contact with them. For patients, this means the drugs are strong enough to damage or kill cancer cells. But this also means the drugs can be a concern for others who might be exposed to them. This is why there are safety rules and recommendations for people who handle chemo drugs."

Further, "It's important to know that not all medicines and drugs to treat cancer work the same way or have the same safety precautions. The information below describes some safety concerns of traditional or standard chemotherapy." The ACS further advises:

- Special clothing will be worn by health care professionals who administer infusion chemotherapy, including a special protective gown, two pairs of gloves, and a face shield.

- Any spilled IV chemo, any powder or dust from a pill or capsule, or any liquid from oral or other kinds of chemo can be hazardous to others if they are around it.

- It generally takes about 48 to 72 hours for your body to break down and/or get rid of most chemo drugs. But it's important to know that each chemo drug is excreted or passed through the body a bit differently. Some drugs take longer to leave your body.

- Most of the drug waste comes out in your body fluids, such as urine, stool, tears, sweat, and vomit.

- When chemo drugs or their waste are outside your body, they can harm or irritate the skin. Other people and pets could be exposed to the drug waste for a few days if they come into contact with any of your body fluids.

- If possible, have children use a different toilet than the one you use.

- Flush the toilet twice after you use it. Put the lid down before flushing to avoid splashing. If possible, you may want to use a separate toilet during this time. If this is not possible, wear gloves to clean the toilet seat after each use.

- Sit on the toilet when you use it to cut down on splashing.

- Keep the toilet lid down when you're not using it to keep pets from drinking the water.

- Always wash your hands with warm water and soap after using the toilet. Dry your hands with paper towels and throw them away.

- If you vomit into the toilet, clean off all splashes and flush twice. If you vomit into a bucket or basin, carefully empty it into the toilet without splashing the contents and flush twice. Wash out the bucket with hot, soapy water and rinse it; empty the wash and rinse water into the toilet, then flush. Dry the bucket with paper towels and throw them away.

- Caregivers (e.g., family members) should wear 2 pairs of throw-away gloves if they need to touch any of your body fluids.

- Any clothes or sheets that have body fluids on them should be washed in your washing machine – not by hand. Wash them in warm water with regular laundry detergent. Do not wash them with other clothes. If they can't be washed right away, seal them in a plastic bag.

> No doubt you are aware that we are regularly exposed to a variety of chemicals in the environment that are harmful, including some that are linked to cancer.[158, 159] You may not know, however, that many pharmaceutical drugs are also making their way into the environment daily, including into our water supplies.

Part of the reason for this contamination by pharmaceuticals is that people continue to dispose of unused drugs by flushing them down the toilet – in fact, patients are advised to do so under certain conditions.[160] Although some maintain that there is no evidence that small amounts of drugs in the water supply present a problem, it is apparently true that no one really knows. As Harvard Health Publishing notes[161],

- Pharmaceutical pollution doesn't seem to be harming humans yet, but disturbing clues from aquatic life suggest now is the time for preventive action.
- Water quality experts and environmental advocates are increasingly concerned about another kind of water pollution: chemicals from prescription drugs and over-the-counter medications that get into lakes, rivers, and streams.

Rather than flushing drugs into the water supply, I urge you to look for drug take-back programs in your community or to search for disposal locations on the Drug Enforcement Administration Division Control Division website[162] (link is provided under Suggested Resources in the Appendices section).

Another reason that drugs make their way into the water supply is that they are not fully used (*metabolized*) by our bodies. Consequently, excess drugs are contained in the patient's urine, feces, and sweat. As Harvard Health Publishing notes[163],

- The typical American medicine cabinet is full of unused and expired drugs, only a fraction of which get disposed of properly. Data collected from a medication collection program in California in 2007 suggest that about half of all medications – both prescription and over-the-counter – are discarded. That's probably a high-end estimate, but even if the real proportion is lower, there's a lot of unused medication that can potentially get into the water.

- An increasing number of medications are applied as creams or lotions, and the unabsorbed portions of those medications can contribute to the pollution problem when they get washed off. It's been calculated, for example, that one man's use of testosterone cream can wind up putting as much of the hormone into the water as the natural excretions from 300 men.

Interdicting this source of excess drugs is clearly complicated and would require some kind of simple yet reliable collection device. For example, a device that could be added to a conventional toilet to filter out the chemotherapy drugs before they enter the sewage line. Given the potential problem of drug pollution and health, shouldn't interdiction be a high priority for governments around the world?

> Wouldn't it be a sad result if the drugs used to help those in the United States with cancer end up negatively impacting the health of the world, including the promotion of cancers? Such unintended consequences are common occurrences in our increasingly connected world and should not be casually dismissed or ignored.[164]

Other Drugs & Supplements

Pancrelipase

According to Medline Plus[165], Pancrelipase (Creon, Pancreaze, Pertzye, Ultresa, Zenpep) is a delayed-release capsule that

- is used to improve the digestion of food in children and adults who do not have enough pancreatic enzymes that break down food so it can be digested
- used to improve digestion in people who have had surgery to remove all or part of the pancreas or stomach
- acts in place of the enzymes normally made by the pancreas

According to Steven Merlin, the Ultresa brand may not be available in the United States, no generic form of Pancrealipase currently exists and the third most widely prescribed pancrealipase behind Creon and Zenpep is Viokace. (Viokace and Zenpep are products of Nestlé Healthcare Nutrition).

Dexamethasone

Also known by the brand name Decadron®, "Dexamethasone, a corticosteroid, is similar to a natural hormone produced by your adrenal glands. It often is used to replace this chemical when your body does not make enough of it. It relieves inflammation (swelling, heat, redness, and pain) and is used to treat certain forms of arthritis; skin, blood, kidney, eye, thyroid, and intestinal disorders (e.g., colitis); severe allergies; and asthma. Dexamethasone is also used to treat certain types of cancer. Dexamethasone may cause side effects. Tell your doctor if any of these symptoms are severe or do not go away:"[166]

upset stomach	vomiting
dizziness	headache
restlessness	insomnia, anxiety
easy bruising	depression

If you experience any of the following symptoms, call your doctor at once:

skin rash	swollen face, lower legs, or ankles
vision problems	cold or infection that lasts a long time
muscle weakness	black or tarry stool

Prochlorperazine

Also known by the brand name Compazine®, "Prochlorperazine suppositories and tablets are used to control severe nausea and vomiting. Prochlorperazine tablets are also used on a short-term basis to treat anxiety that could not be controlled by other medications."[167]

Potential side effects include but are not limited to, those listed below. Tell your doctor if any of these symptoms are severe or do not go away.

dizziness, feeling unsteady or having trouble keeping your balance	blurred vision
dry mouth	stuffed nose
headache	nausea
constipation	difficulty urinating
widening or narrowing of the pupils (black circles in the center of the eyes)	increased appetite, weight gain
Jitteriness, agitation, difficulty falling asleep or staying asleep	uncontrollable shaking of a part of the body, shuffling walk

Some side effects can be serious. If you experience any of the following symptoms, contact your health care team at once.

fever, sweating, flu-like symptoms	muscle stiffness, neck cramps
falling, confusion	fast or irregular heartbeat
yellowing of the skin or eyes	tightness in the throat
sore throat, chills, and other signs of infection	difficulty breathing or swallowing
uncontrollable, rhythmic face, mouth, or jaw movements	seizures, rash, hives, itching
vision loss, especially at night, seeing everything with a brown tint	swelling of the eyes, face, mouth, lips, tongue, throat, arms, hands, feet, ankles, or lower legs

Ondansetron

Also known by its brand name, Zofran®, "Ondansetron is used to prevent nausea and vomiting caused by cancer chemotherapy, radiation therapy, and surgery. Ondansetron is in a class of medications called serotonin 5-HT3 receptor antagonists. It works by blocking the action of serotonin, a natural substance that may cause nausea and vomiting. Ondansetron may cause side effects. Tell your doctor if any of these symptoms are severe or do not go away:"

headache	constipation
weakness	tiredness
chills	drowsiness

Some side effects can be serious. If you experience any of the following symptoms, call your doctor at once or seek emergency medical treatment:

blurred vision or vision loss	rash, itching, hives, seizures
swelling of the eyes, face, lips, tongue, throat, hands, feet, ankles, or lower legs	difficulty breathing or swallowing, shortness of breath
fast, slow, or irregular heartbeat, chest pain	hoarseness
hallucinations (seeing things or hearing voices that do not exist)	dizziness, light-headedness, or fainting
nausea, vomiting, or diarrhea	agitation, confusion
stiff or twitching muscles, loss of coordination	fever, excessive sweating

Docusate and Senna

A combination of two agents known by the brand name Senokot-S®, "Senna is the fruit (pod) or leaf of the plant Senna Alexandrina. It is approved in the US as a laxative for short-term treatment of constipation. Senna contains many chemicals called sennosides. Sennosides irritate the lining of the bowel, which causes a laxative effect. Senna is an FDA-approved over-the-counter (OTC) laxative. It is used to treat constipation and also to clear the bowel before procedures such as colonoscopy."[168]

Docusate is a stool softener. "Stool softeners are used on a short-term basis to relieve constipation by people who should avoid straining during bowel movements because of heart conditions, hemorrhoids, and other problems. They work by softening stools to make them easier to pass."[169]

Esomeprazole

Esomeprasole is available in both prescription and nonprescription forms (e.g., Nexium®), "Nonprescription (over the counter) esomeprazole is used to treat frequent heartburn (heartburn that occurs at least 2 or more days a week) in adults. Esomeprazole is in a class of medications called proton pump inhibitors (PPI). It works by decreasing the amount of acid made in the stomach."[170]

Hydromorphone

Also known by the brand name Dilaudid®, "Hydromorphone is used to relieve pain. "Hydromorphone is in a class of medications called opiate (narcotic) analgesics. It works by changing the way the brain and nervous system respond to pain. Hydromorphone may be habit forming, especially with prolonged use. Take hydromorphone exactly as directed."[171]

Pegfilgrastim-bmez

According to Mayo Clinic[172],

- Pegfilgrastim-bmez injections are used to treat neutropenia (low white blood cells) that is caused by cancer medicines.
- It is a synthetic (man-made) form of a substance that is naturally produced in your body called a colony-stimulating factor.
- Pegfilgrastim-bmez helps the bone marrow to make new white blood cells.
- When certain cancer medicines are used to fight cancer cells, they also affect the white blood cells that fight infections.
- Pegfilgrastim-bmez is used to reduce the risk of infection[173] while you are being treated with cancer medicines.
- This medicine is available only with your doctor's prescription.

Atropine

Atropine is a drug that is used for a variety of reasons, including as a smooth muscle relaxant, to reduce secretions, and for chemotherapy-induced diarrhea (CID). "(CID) is a predictable yet undertreated side effect of several frequently used chemotherapy agents and can lead to delays in treatment and poor quality of life."[174]

Pantoprazole

According to Medline Plus,[175]

- Pantoprazole is used to treat damage from gastroesophageal reflux disease (GERD), a condition in which the backward flow of acid from the stomach causes heartburn and possible injury to the esophagus (the tube between the throat and stomach).

- Pantoprazole is used to allow the esophagus to heal and prevent further damage to the esophagus in adults with GERD.
- Pantoprazole is in a class of medications called proton-pump inhibitors. It works by decreasing the amount of acid made in the stomach.

Potassium

According to WebMD[176],

- Potassium is a mineral that's crucial for life. Potassium is necessary for the heart, kidneys, and other organs to work normally.
- Most people who eat a healthy diet should get enough potassium naturally. Low potassium is associated with a risk of high blood pressure, heart disease, stroke, arthritis, cancer, digestive disorders, and infertility. For people with low potassium, doctors sometimes recommend improved diets -- or potassium supplements -- to prevent or treat some of these conditions.
- Potassium deficiencies are more common in people who:
  o Use certain medicines, such as diuretics
  o Have physically demanding jobs
  o Athletes exercising in hot climates and sweating excessively
  o Have health conditions that affect their digestive absorption, such as Crohn's disease
  o Have an eating disorder
  o Smoke
  o Abuse of alcohol or drugs
  o Always take potassium supplements with a full glass of water or juice.
- Good natural food sources of potassium include:
  o Bananas
  o Avocados
  o Peanuts and tree nuts such as almonds, pecans, and walnuts
  o Citrus fruits
  o Leafy, green vegetables
  o Milk
  o Potatoes

o Keep in mind that some types of cooking, such as boiling, can decrease the potassium content in some foods.

As with any drug or supplement, always follow your physician's orders, do not take more potassium than prescribed, and always contact your health care team with questions and do so immediately if you experience side effects (e.g., upset stomach, allergic reaction, muscle weakness, confusion, tingling sensation in the limbs, low blood pressure).

Boost® Nutritional Drink[177]

Unintentional weight loss is common in cancer and various nutritional drinks for weight gain are available on the market. The Boost brand is popular and offers several different versions, including Boost Plus® which supplies 360 calories per 8-ounce serving, and Boost® Very High Calorie provides 530 calories per 8-ounce serving.

The brand also offers "Boost® Soothe Drink developed in collaboration with oncology centers and patients and is designed to provide nutritional support for those experiencing certain side effects of cancer treatment, such as taste changes and oral discomfort. It provides a cooling and soothing effect plus 300 calories to help gain or maintain weight, with 10 g of high-quality protein to help maintain muscle. BOOST® Soothe Drink is formulated without certain vitamins and minerals known to have a metallic aftertaste and contains no artificial sweeteners, flavors, or colors."[178]

Enterade® Nutritional Drink

Enterade is a new, non-prescriptive nutritional drink that the manufacturer claims, is "The first plant-based medical food that is clinically proven to help reduce the GI side effects of chemotherapy, radiation treatment, and immunotherapy."

Some patients who have used Enterade find the taste more appealing and less sweet than Ensure® and Boost®. I've just started using the product and so can't offer an opinion based on experience at this time.

Note that as of the time I'm writing this, the manufacturer acknowledges that their claims have not been evaluated by the FDA. The product website, however, offers more information, including the results of clinical studies - https://enterade.com

Suggested Resources

Cancer Information

- **Pancreatic Cancer Action Network**, https://www.pancan.org/
- **Cancer Research UK**, https://www.cancerresearchuk.org/
- **The National Pancreatic Cancer Foundation** - https://pancreasfoundation.org/
- **NIH Clinical Trials**, a database of privately and publicly funded clinical studies conducted around the world - https://www.clinicaltrials.gov/
- **National Cancer Institute** – https://www.cancer.gov
- **Cancer Connect**, a support group - https://news.cancerconnect.com/
- **Belong**, a support group - https://cancer.belong.life/
- **Road to Recovery**, American Cancer Society transportation program - https://www.cancer.org/support-programs-and-services/road-to-recovery.html
- **Let's Win! Pancreatic Cancer**, breaking research, results of clinical trial studies written for the lay person, practical information, and survivor stories and videos - https://letswinpc.org/
- **Seena Magowitz Foundation**, inspirational survivor stories, articles, and webinars by pancreatic cancer surgeons and oncologists - https://seenamagowitzfoundation.org/
- **The Hirshberg Foundation for Pancreatic Cancer Research**, https://pancreatic.org/pancreatic-cancer/about-the-pancreas/the-pancreas/

Planning Information

- **Mayo Clinic**, https://www.mayoclinic.org/healthy-lifestyle/consumer-health/in-depth/living-wills/art-20046303
- **The National Institute on Aging**, https://www.nia.nih.gov/health/advance-care-planning-health-care-directives
- **The Family Care Alliance**, https://www.caregiver.org/resource/advance-health-care-directives-and-polst/

Other

- **A PC Magazine review of the best password managers for 2022**, https://www.pcmag.com/picks/the-best-password-managers
- **Zoom Conferencing**, https://zoom.us
- **National Library of Medicine Medline Plus** - https://medlineplus.gov/
- **Disability Placards & Plates**, NC DMV - https://bit.ly/3bbIfwv

- **Controlled Substance Public Disposal Locations** -
  https://bit.ly/3QqO60i

The Doughnut Hole

What is the "doughnut hole?" According to Healthcare.gov,

> "Most plans with Medicare prescription drug coverage
> (Part D) have a coverage gap (called a "doughnut hole").
> This means that after you and your drug plan have spent
> a certain amount of money for covered drugs, you have
> to pay all costs out-of-pocket for your prescriptions up to
> a yearly limit. Once you have spent up to the yearly limit,
> your coverage gap ends and your drug plan helps pay for
> covered drugs again."[179]

An example of the doughnut hole is the cost of the Creon® enzyme
that people with pancreatic cancer are prescribed. According to Arjun
Gupta, MD, an oncology fellow at Johns Hopkins Sidney Kimmel
Comprehensive Cancer Center, Baltimore, Maryland[180]:

- Pancreatic enzyme replacement therapy (PERT) is often an essential
  component of the treatment regimen for patients with pancreatic
  cancer, but it can be very pricey
- Out-of-pocket costs for a 30-day supply of enzymes for Medicare
  beneficiaries can be as high as $1000
- This (cost) can contribute to financial toxicity for patients who
  already have a high symptom burden and distress. The high cost of
  this supportive care has been underappreciated
- Out-of-pocket costs for two large pancreas enzyme capsules, which
  are often required for a meal, may be $15. And these need to be
  taken at every meal and may be more expensive than the meal itself
- Among Medicare beneficiaries, the expected out-of-pocket costs for
  a 30-day supply of optimally dosed PERT averaged $999 across
  formulations. Patients' costs, including deductibles and coinsurance,
  ranged from $853 to $1536

- The out-of-pocket costs were lower after patients met the deductible ($673; range, $527 to $1210) and continued to decrease after reaching catastrophic coverage ($135; range, $105 to $242)

- There has been a lot of publicity about very expensive anticancer drugs, but little has been said about the costs of products used in supportive care

- While it's true that many patients cannot afford the drugs, there are patient-assistance programs where they can often get them free of charge. But supportive care agents, such as those for constipation or enzymes – all of those can nickel-and-dime you and end up being very costly.

- These agents add substantially to the drug cost burden. Some patients also need insulin, which is also insanely expensive

- One of the reasons for the high cost of PERT is that there are very few options, and all the available products are brand-name agents.

- Clinicians often under prescribe pancreatic enzymes in clinical practice.

- Gupta and colleagues assessed PERT costs using the Medicare Part D formulary and pricing files for the first quarter of 2020. Point-of-sale and out-of-pocket costs for each PERT formulation were calculated among Part D stand-alone and Medicare Advantage prescription drug plans.

- Costs were then assessed using three scenarios: the standard benefit design, with a $435 deductible and 25% coinsurance after the deductible is met; 25% coinsurance to fill a prescription after the deductible while in the coverage gap until the patient spends $6,350 out of pocket, and 5% coinsurance once catastrophic coverage is reached.

- Across 3,974 plans nationwide, four formulations in 17 different doses were covered by Medicare plans during the study period. Doses ranged from 3000 to 40,000 lipase units, and the per-unit list price ranged from $1.44 to $13.89.

- The point-of-sale price for a 30-day supply of optimally dosed PERT ranged from $2,109 to $4,840.

- Gupta noted that a "good-sized meal often requires 80,000 units of lipase or two of the very largest pills. Of note, these pills need to be taken meal after meal every meal throughout a patient's life."

- Prescribers and dieticians try to find the least expensive options, including patient-assistance programs, but in the end, they are sometimes forced to under prescribe. Some patients will go and buy over-the-counter pancreatic enzyme supplements, and it seems like a good way to cut costs, but it is not recommended for people with pancreatic cancer."
- The problem with these over the counter formulations is that they are not regulated. The enzyme content in them is also minuscule, in the range of hundreds of units instead of the 50,000 units needed per meal. Patients end up spending much more on ineffective therapies.

When I first started my therapy, I was not prescribed Creon. It was after I experienced the lightening of stool and darkening of urine that I was prescribed two 36,000-unit Creon capsules with each meal. We first filled my prescriptions at CVS with a co-pay cost of $567 for 180 capsules (a 30-day supply). Diane learned that CVS was not a designated provider under our supplemental insurance policy and so the cost could be lower elsewhere.

It turned out that the local Publix pharmacy was a designated provider and by moving from CVS to Publix we were able to reduce the cost to $368. However, on the second prescription filled at Publix, the cost rose to $546 thanks to the doughnut hole effect. To get the lower price, we will have to first exceed prescription payments of all drugs, including Creon, by about $2,500.

About halfway into my chemotherapy, I again occasionally experienced light-colored stool. I was instructed to take three Creon capsules before every meal and that additional capsule did seem to do the trick. At the same time, that additional capsule means that a prescription that used to last for 30 days now lasts just 20 days. When my Creon prescription is $546 the cost of one Creon capsule is about $3 and the daily cost of nine Creon capsules (three capsules per meal) is about $27. I may need to increase my Creon dose further at some point and to take Creon for the rest of my life. So, Creon will be a significant cost of my care for us.

> As an aside, the co-pay for a morphine pill that I was prescribed was $0.58 for 30 pills. Apparently, the cost of opioids like morphine is low due to generics.[181] I see no

reason the same kind of price decrease shouldn't happen when generic forms of enzymes like Creon become available. In the meantime, however, patients needing enzyme supplements may have little choice but to pay the high cost of enzyme brands to survive.

We asked our health care team about non-prescription enzyme alternatives to Creon like *Vital Nutrients Pancreatic Enzymes*. After checking the ingredients which appeared to be nearly identical to Creon, we were advised that I would have to take two of the non-prescriptive enzymes for every one Creon capsule.

Although the cost of the non-prescriptive enzyme is much lower than Creon – $39 for 90 capsules on Amazon[182], a bottle would last me only 10 days. We've decided to stick with Creon which seems to work well for me and exit the doughnut hole sooner than later so insurance picks up more of the cost.

The National Council on Aging offers suggestions to avoid the doughnut hole, including:[183]

- **State Pharmaceutical Assistance Program (SPAP)**: Some, but not all, states have a SPAP to help people pay for their medications. Sometimes the SPAP will contribute an amount toward your Part D premium, or it may work to offset your prescription costs.
- **Patient Assistance Programs**: Brand-name drug manufacturers often have these programs to provide discounts or no-cost medications to those who qualify. You may have to provide proof of income and spending on the prescription to be able to take advantage of these programs.
- **Disease Funds**: Disease funds are supported by charitable groups and help to pay for medications and treatments for a specific disease or condition.
- **Generics**: Talk to your doctor about whether any generics may be a good substitute for expensive brand-name drugs. If your medication is in a higher cost tier or not covered on your plan's formulary (approved drug list), you may want to see if you can ask for an exception to get the plan to cover it completely or at a lower cost.

- **"Best" Price**: Another strategy is to ask your pharmacist for the "best" price for the prescription. Sometimes costs for drugs may be less if you do not use your insurance. Be mindful that any drug you purchase outside of your insurance will not automatically count toward satisfying your deductible or getting you out of the doughnut hole. Contact your plan to determine if the drug purchases you made outside of your Part D plan can be counted toward your true out-of-pocket costs and/or are eligible for reimbursement.

Home vs Hospital Injection

I mentioned under My Cancer Journey an injection that I receive a couple of days after home infusion to address low white blood cell counts. We return to the hospital to receive this injection, primarily for cost considerations.

Diane is a registered nurse and could easily give me the injection in our home but doing so would rely on our supplemental insurance which has a co-pay of about $1,800 per shot. I started receiving this injection on my second cycle of therapy so getting the shot for the eleven remaining cycles would mean a $19,800 cost, depending upon the doughnut effect.

Getting the injection at the hospital, which requires that we make an hour round trip to Durham, check in, and then wait for a five-minute procedure, ensures that the cost of the injection is covered under Medicare part B. Perhaps you will agree that this is yet another *nutty* situation in America's baffling healthcare system.

The True Price of Cancer Treatment

I was curious to know the cost of my treatment at the halfway mark, so I did a quick tally of Medicare claims related to my treatment. The total was about $220,700 which included special procedures like my bile duct stent. Assuming that the remainder of my treatments includes just the chemotherapy and injection for white blood cells, we're probably looking at an additional $82,000 – for a total six month therapy cost of $302,700. Of course, there are other costs such as Creon and other drugs that I take at home. It's no wonder that a cancer diagnosis can upend the patient and her family, even if she has insurance. Studies have found that cancer patients:[184]

- Were 71% more likely than Americans without the disease to have bills in collections, face tax liens and mortgage foreclosure, or experience other financial setbacks.
- Were 2½ times more likely to declare bankruptcy than those without the disease, and patients who went bankrupt were more likely to die than those who did not. Oncologists have a name for this: "financial toxicity"

The true price of cancer is clearly not just the cost of treatment, but also the impact the treatment costs can have on the cancer patient and her family.

The Very Long Road to New Drug Therapies

To see a headline like, "Hitting Rewind on the Spread of Pancreatic Cancer"[185] you might think that a new and effective therapy is now available for pancreatic cancer patients. Unfortunately, such eyeball-grabbing headlines can be misleading and do not reflect the full story.

Regarding the headline above, the full article was an interview with a researcher whose research suggested the possibility that therapy could be developed to "reverse aggressive cancer cells back to less aggressive ones and therefore make the tumors much more treatable with standard therapy." So, while the research finding is interesting and encouraging, an actual therapy based on the research is many years into the future.

What does it take to move from a research idea to a drug that is approved by FDA? There are five steps to the Drug Development Process[186]:

1. **Discovery and Development**: Research for a new drug begins in the laboratory.
2. **Preclinical Research**: Drugs undergo laboratory and animal testing to answer basic questions about safety.
3. **Clinical Research**: Drugs are tested on people to make sure they are safe and effective.

4. **FDA Review**: FDA review teams thoroughly examine all of the submitted data related to the drug or device and make a decision to approve or not to approve it.
5. **FDA Post-Market Safety Monitoring**: FDA monitors all drug and device safety once products are available for use by the public.

Referring to the headline above, the research was apparently in the early phase of the Discovery and Development step. The research incorporated "genetic mouse models for pancreatic cancer and mini tumors" – a typical early step but well in advance of any use in humans.

During the Preclinical Research step, a comprehensive and formal test plan needs to be established. The tests may be conducted *in vitro* (in a test tube) or *in vivo* (in a living organism like a mouse). FDA notes, "Usually, preclinical studies are not very large. However, these studies must provide detailed information on dosing and toxicity levels. After preclinical testing, researchers review their findings and decide whether the drug should be tested in people."

Assuming the Preclinical Research does not reveal safety problems, the Clinical Research step may be started. FDA notes, "While preclinical research answers basic questions about a drug's safety, it is not a substitute for studies of ways the drug will interact with the human body. 'Clinical research' refers to studies, or trials, that are done in people."

A more advanced protocol must be developed for Clinical Research trials that answers numerous questions from who qualifies to participate in the study, to how the data will be reviewed and analyzed. Multiple trials are conducted with an increasing number of participants through four phases:

Phase	Study Participants	Length of Study	Purpose	Typical Outcome
1	20 to 100 healthy volunteers or people with the disease/condition.	Several months	Safety and dosage	Approximately 70% of drugs move to the next phase

	Study Participants	Length of Study	Purpose	
2	Study Participants: Up to several hundred people with the disease/condition.	Length of Study: Several months to 2 years	Purpose: Efficacy and side effects	Approximately 33% of drugs move to the next phase
3	300 to 3,000 volunteers who have the disease or condition	1 to 4 years	Efficacy and monitoring of adverse reactions	Approximately 25-30% of drugs move to the next phase
4	Several thousand volunteers who have the disease/condition	Safety and efficacy	Examine long-term effectiveness and adverse effects after FDA approval.	

Note that many potential drug therapies fail to make it through the four phases outlined above. Further, for drugs that do make it to the fourth phase, it is easily a journey of 5-years or longer. Note, too, that patients who participate in early phase drug clinical trials are exposing themselves to potential side effects of the new therapy under investigation – some of which can be severe or fatal.[187] There may also be costs incurred by clinical trial participants that aren't covered by the drug company or insurance.

FDA notes that for drugs that make it through the trial phases, "If a drug developer has evidence from its early tests and preclinical and clinical research that a drug is safe and effective for its intended use, the company can file an application to market the drug. The FDA review team thoroughly examines all submitted data on the drug and makes a decision to approve or not to approve it."

In Step 4 of the Drug Development Process companies submit a New Drug Application (NDA) to FDA and,

> "If it is complete, the review team has 6 to 10 months to make a decision on whether to approve the drug… Often, though, remaining issues need to be resolved

before the drug can be approved for marketing. Sometimes FDA requires the developer to address questions based on existing data. In other cases, FDA requires additional studies. At this point, the developer can decide whether or not to continue further development. If a developer disagrees with an FDA decision, there are mechanisms for formal appeal."

So, to the 5-year plus window to complete the four phases of drug trials, add at least a year or more until a drug receives FDA approval. Regarding Step 5 of the Drug Development Process FDA notes,

"Even though clinical trials provide important information on a drug's efficacy and safety, it is impossible to have complete information about the safety of a drug at the time of approval. Despite the rigorous steps in the process of drug development, limitations exist. Therefore, the true picture of a product's safety actually evolves over the months and even years that make up a product's lifetime in the marketplace. FDA reviews reports of problems with prescription and over-the-counter drugs, and can decide to add cautions to the dosage or usage information, as well as other measures for more serious issues."

It is important to recognize that, although a relatively rare event, drugs approved by FDA have been later recalled due to hazards that revealed themselves only after the drug was in wide use. Some of these more recent recalls include Bextra®, Cylert®, Vioxx®, Meridia®, and Raptiva®.[188]

The takeaway is that you shouldn't be fooled by "breakthrough" headlines – new drug development is a lengthy and uncertain journey. If you do find a clinical trial for which you qualify, then I urge you to ensure that you fully understand the informed consent document which includes potential risks and non-covered costs.[189]

A Peek Through the Keyhole

As I noted in the Preface, I am a private person by nature. By contrast, Diane is very outgoing. So, I want to give you a peek into our lives through the images below to give you a sense of who we are.

Diane and Bob

Diane and I decided to get married on Halloween, which is also Diane's birthday – this may have been her idea to make it easy for me to remember our wedding and her birthday. We held the wedding ceremony at our nearly one-hundred-year-old NJ home, and all attendees dressed in costume, including our daughter who officiated.

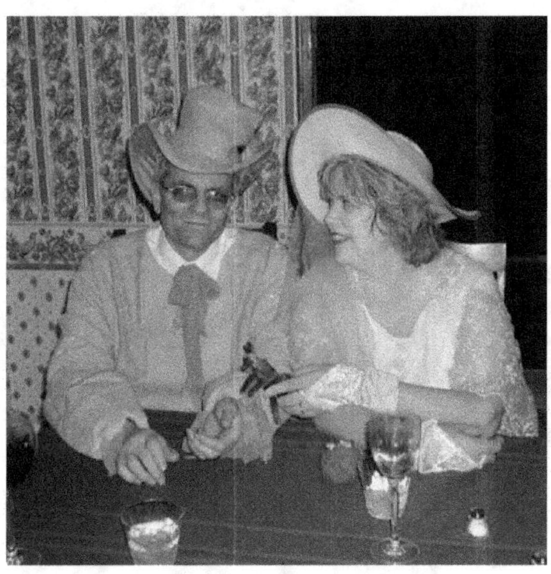

Having a few drinks too many, I fell asleep and awoke before sun up to an empty house except for our old rescue dog, Sandy, who was staring at me. I grabbed a leash and Sandy and I headed out for a walk around the block as dawn approached. I wondered why cars were slowing down to nearly a stop until I realized that I was still wearing my ghost costume.

Diane's Art

When Diane and I moved to NC from NJ, several items were lost along the way, including a still life[190] poster we bought while in Sweden. The painting below is Diane's second attempt at painting anything and is a faithful reproduction of that lost poster. Diane continues expanding her art with other themes and methods.

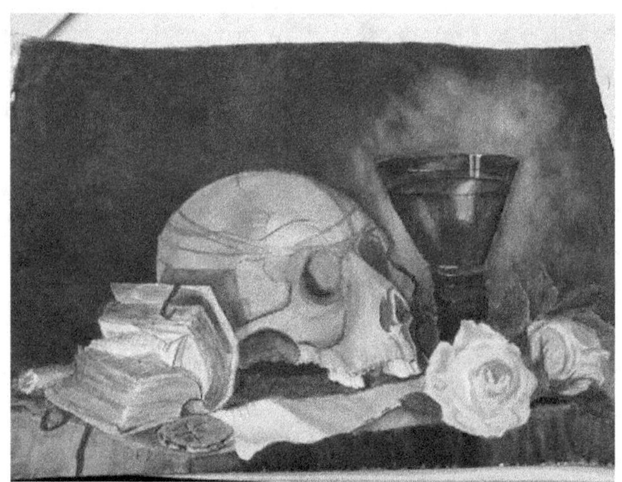

Still Life

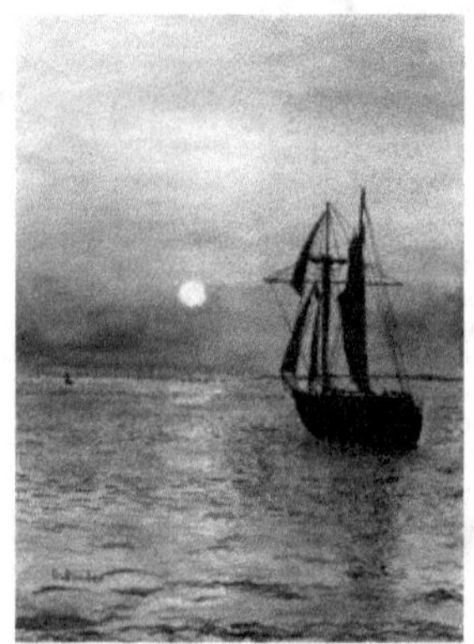
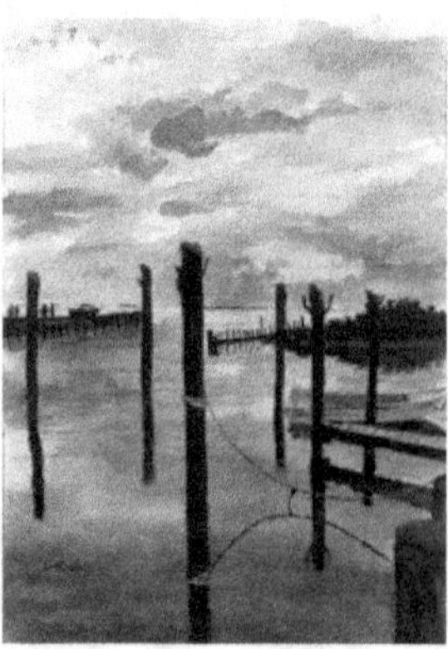
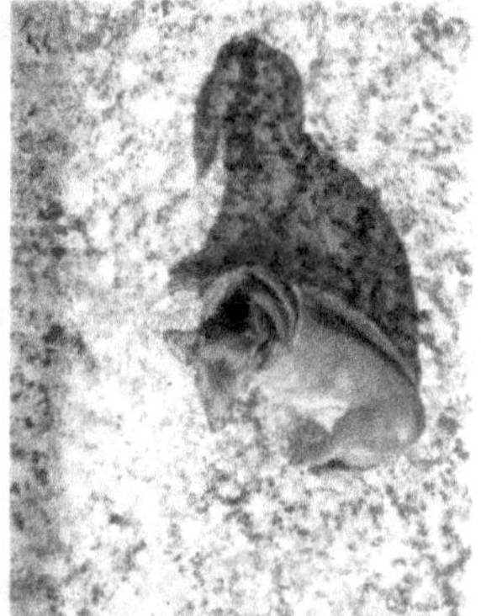

See https://geogalleries.com/Paintings_by_Diane

Bob's Hikes

When I was a kid, my father would wake me at o'dark early on winter weekends to go hunting. As I got dressed, he'd pack us a simple lunch of sandwiches, fruit, and a thermos of Eight O'Clock coffee. We'd load the dog and shotguns into the car, and head out to be in the woods at daybreak when hunting started. We'd walk for miles through woods and corn fields until dusk, often times through snow or rain, taking breaks for warm coffee and our lunch. Occasionally, we'd take small game, too: rabbits, ring-necked pheasants, grouse, and squirrels. My mother would later prepare our bounty by roasting some and turning others into meat pies.

I was never a fan of hunting. I liked seeing the game as they were flushed by our dog's expert nose and baying, but I had no interest in killing anything. Just before starting high school, I reluctantly told my father that I didn't want to hunt anymore. He seemed confused and maybe a little hurt, but he didn't insist that I continue and we never discussed it further.

While going through a midlife crisis as I approached forty, I was fortunate to meet another Bob at my new job. Bob had a similar non-lethal view of the woods, and he quickly became a big brother to me. We spent countless hours traipsing through the woods as trail maintainers for the NY/NJ Trail Conference[191], members of New Jersey Search and Rescue (NJSAR)[192], hiking, biking, and cross-country skiing. Diane has her art; I have my hikes.

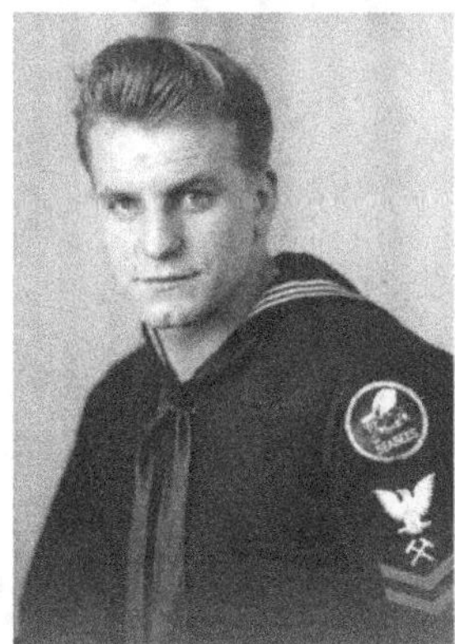
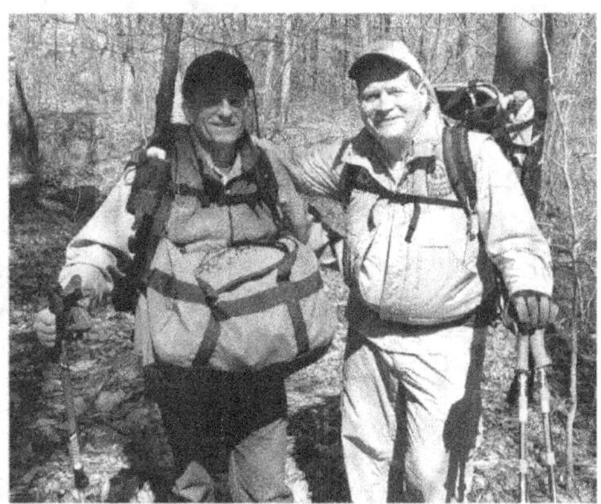

My father in his service uniform; the "Bobs" on the trail

Our Canine Companions

Over the years, we have taken in shelter dogs, some of whom were treated badly in their former lives, but all worth saving. They enriched our daily lives and took a piece of our hearts with them when they departed.

Buster

Buster was a Schipperke, also known in Belgium as the "little captain" who is often found on barges. Buster did not suffer fools kindly and was Diane's loyal defender. With his thick coat of fur, Buster loved resting in the snow and watching the world go by.

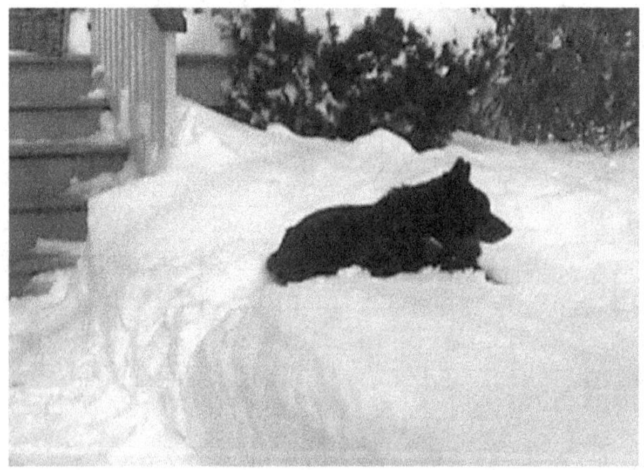

Sandy

After Buster's departure, Diane wanted to help another rescue and asked our vet if he knew about any dogs that nobody else wanted. Sandy was that "junkyard dog," old and flea-bitten, anemic, and in heart failure. His health limited him to the first floor of the house, and many nights Diane would sleep on the sofa with Sandy next to her in his bed so she could keep watch over him. His time with us was short but it had to be the best few months of his hard life.

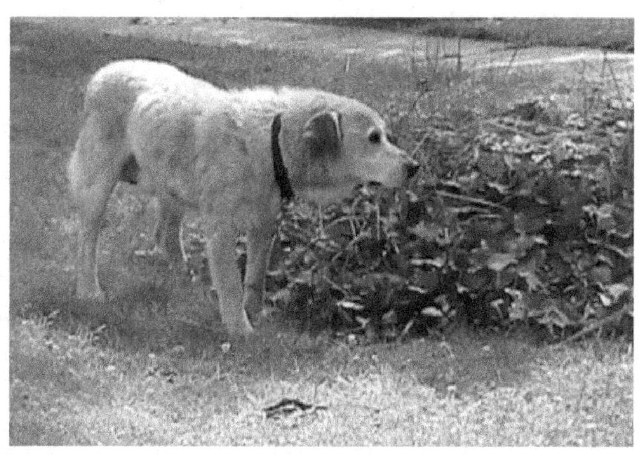

Killian and Shorty

After Sandy's departure, Shorty (left) and Killian (right) joined us. Killian was an extremely skittish dog who cowered at the sound of a bouncing basketball and the crack of thunder. Our vet also thought he may have been shot in the head by a pellet gun. Shorty was jovial and trusting and seemed to have a calming effect on Killian. As we were preparing for our move to NC, a tumor was discovered in Shorty, and he did not make the trip with us. Killian developed dementia after we arrived in NC where he made his departure.

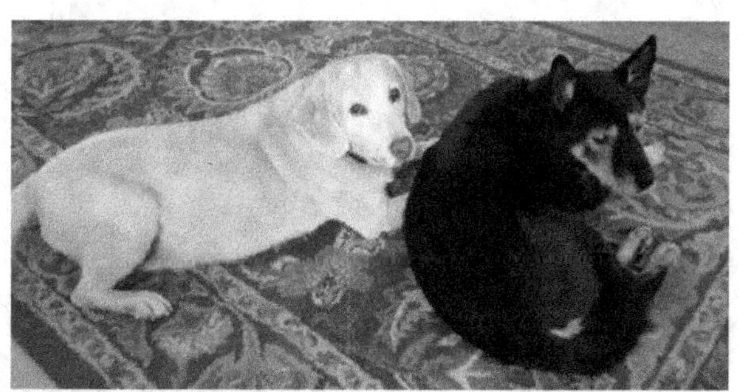

Ozzie

Ozzie is our current canine companion. We welcomed him while still living in NJ and he quickly became the youthful companion to Killian and Shorty. As a child, Diane had a dachshund, but the breed was new to me – meaning I didn't understand how energetic and stubborn dachshunds can be. I've yet to meet a dachshund owner who claimed to be able to train their dog past a few simple commands. Oz can be a royal pain when he gets rambunctious, but we wouldn't trade him for anything in the world. Below is Oz with one of his many toys, and Oz posing on Diane's shoulder.

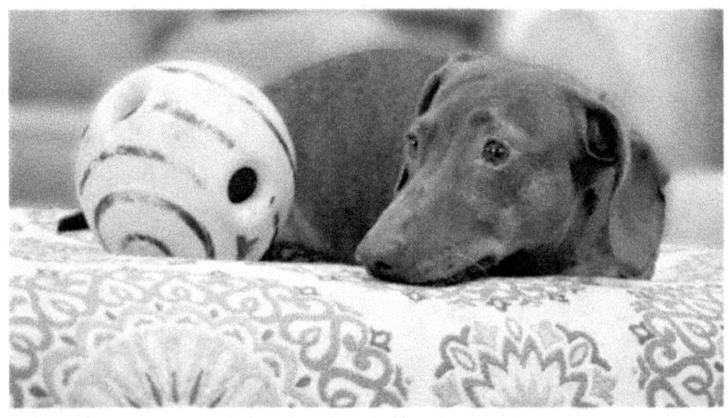

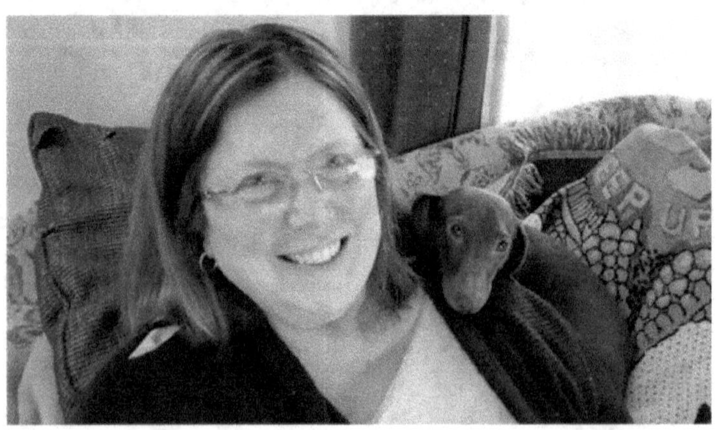

GLOSSARY

The terms contained in this glossary were excerpted and merged from several online sources, including:

1. Johns Hopkins Medicine Pathology - https://pathology.jhu.edu/pancreas/glossary
2. Pancreatic Cancer Action Network - https://pancan.org/facing-pancreatic-cancer/about-pancreatic-cancer/glossary-of-terms/
3. Hirshberg Foundation for Pancreatic Cancer Research - https://pancreatic.org/pancreatic-cancer/glossary-of-terms/
4. Let's Win! Pancreatic Cancer - https://letswinpc.org/glossary/

Note that the websites above may offer different definitions of terms and update their information from time to time. Refer to the referenced website for the most current information.

Term	Definition	Ref
5-FU (5-fluorouracil)	A chemotherapeutic drug commonly used to treat pancreatic cancer.	1
Abdomen	The belly: the part of the body that contains all of the structures between the chest and pelvis.	4
Abraxane (paclitaxel)	One of the approved chemotherapy drugs for pancreatic cancer, it inhibits cell division and promotes cell death. It is often given with gemcitabine.	4
ABRAXANE® (albumin-bound paclitaxel):	A chemotherapy drug approved by the FDA in 2013 to treat metastatic pancreatic adenocarcinoma in combination with gemcitabine (Gemzar®). ABRAXANE is a modified form of the chemotherapy drug paclitaxel.	2

Term	Definition	Ref
Abscess	A pus-filled cavity. Usually caused by an infection.	1
Acinar cells	Special cells in the pancreas that produce digestive enzymes.	4
Acquired mutations	Genetic changes that develop during a person's lifetime, either as a random error made in DNA copying or as a result of harmful environmental factors.	4
Acupuncture	Practice of inserting needles through the skin into specific points on the body to reduce pain or induce anesthesia.	4
Acute pain	Sudden, short-lived pain that subsides when healing occurs.	4
Adenocarcinoma	Cancer that begins with cells that line certain internal organs and have gland-like properties.	4
Adenoma	Benign tumor of epithelial tissue with glandular origin, glandular characteristics, or both. Adenomas can grow from many glandular organs, including the adrenal glands, pituitary gland, thyroid, prostate, and others. Although adenomas are benign, over time they may transform to become malignant, at which point they are called adenocarcinomas.	3
Adjuvant chemotherapy	Adjuvant chemotherapy is given after a pancreatic tumor is removed with surgery to prevent the cancer from coming back.	3
Adjuvant drug	A drug that, when added to another drug speeds or improves its effect.	4
Adjuvant therapy	A treatment given after surgery.	4

Term	Definition	Ref
Advance directives	Documents involved in a patient's healthcare that allow others to know which types of care that patient wants and does not want, or to determine who will make medical decisions if the patient cannot do so.	4
Adverse Event	A health-related problem that occurs during treatment that may or may not be related to the treatment. Adverse events may be mild, moderate, or severe. All adverse events must be reported to the Food and Drug Administration (FDA).	2
Afinitor (everolimus)	An approved antineoplastic chemotherapy drug used to treat pancreatic neuroendocrine tumors.	4
Alcohol nerve block	Procedure in which a local anesthetic is injected into the nerve root of the celiac plexus using guidance by ultrasonography or computed tomography to produce numbness or reduce pain.	4
Alternative Therapy	A type of treatment not regulated by the U.S. FDA because they are unproven and often promoted as cures. Alternative therapies include treatment through the use of dietary supplements, special teas, vitamins, herbal preparations, and practices such as massage therapy, acupuncture, spiritual healing, and meditation.	2
Ambulatory Surgery Center	A facility that provides minimally invasive surgeries on an out-patient basis. Most ambulatory surgeries require patients to stay at the center for 2-4 hours.	2
Ampulla of Vater	Enlargement of the ducts from the liver and pancreas at the point where they enter the small intestine; bile from the liver and secretions from the pancreas come through	4

Term	Definition	Ref
	the Ampulla of Vater to mix with food in the duodenum and aid digestion.	
Amylase	An enzyme secreted in saliva and by the pancreas that breaks down starch (complex carbohydrates).	2
Analgesic	A drug that reduces pain: acetaminophen, ibuprofen, and aspirin are analgesics.	4
Anastomosis	A surgical joining of two hollow structures. It is similar to attaching two ends of a garden hose. For example, a gastrojejunostomy is a surgical procedure that connects the stomach and the jejunum (small intestine.)	1
Anemia	The condition of having a lower-than-normal number of red blood cells or quantity of hemoglobin. Anemia diminishes the capacity of the blood to carry oxygen.	4
Anesthesia	The loss of feeling or awareness caused by drugs. Local anesthesia causes loss of feeling in a part of the body. General anesthesia puts the person to sleep.	2
Angiogenesis	Formation of new blood vessels; some cancer treatments work by blocking angiogenesis, called antiangiogenesis, with the goal of slowing or preventing tumor growth.	4
Angiography	A radiographic technique used to visualize blood vessels. A contrast medium (a dye) is usually injected into the vessels to make them appear white on the x-rays.	1
Anorexia	A condition marked by a diminished appetite and aversion to food. Patients with advanced cancer may have anorexia-related	4

Term	Definition	Ref
	weight loss or wasting.	
Antibody	Proteins in the plasma and serum of the immune system that help the body fight infections. Also called immunoglobulin.	4
Anticoagulant	A drug that thins the blood to reduce the risk of blood clots.	4
Anticonvulsants	Drugs used to prevent or treat seizures; they may also be used to enhance the effect of pain medications.	4
Antidepressants	Drugs used to treat depression; they may also be used to enhance the effect of pain medications.	4
Antiemetics	Drugs that help to prevent and control nausea and vomiting.	4
Antigen	A substance that causes the immune system to make a specific immune response.	2
Antimetabolite	A cancer drug that prevents the "building blocks" of the genetic code from being used.	4
Antioxidants	Human-made or natural substances that may prevent or delay some types of cell damage.	4
Aorta	The large artery that carries oxygen-rich blood from the heart. From the heart it arches backwards and descends into the abdomen where it gives off many branches to supply the organs. The superior mesenteric artery is a major branch of the aorta that can be involved by pancreatic cancer.	1
Ascites	Abnormal buildup of fluid in the belly area	4

Term	Definition	Ref
	(abdomen) or pelvis.	
Asymptomatic	Having no signs or symptoms of disease.	4
Baseline test	A first test, one which future test results are compared to.	4
Benign	Not cancerous; benign tumors do not spread to tissue near them or to other parts of the body.	4
Benign tumors	Tumors which are non-cancerous. These generally grow slowly and do not invade adjacent organs or spread (metastasize) beyond the pancreas.	1
Bile	Fluid made by the liver and stored in the gallbladder; bile is excreted into the small intestine, where it helps digest fat.	4
Bile duct	A tube in the liver through which bile passes.	4
Bilirubin	Dark-green substance formed when red blood cells are broken down. The bilirubin is part of the bile; the abnormal buildup of bilirubin because of an obstruction causes jaundice.	4
Biochemotherapy	Treatment with drugs that boost the body's disease-fighting ability (immunotherapy) and drugs that kill fast-growing cells (chemotherapy).	4
Bioelectromagnetic-based therapy	Involves the use of pulsed energy or magnetic fields to change the body's electromagnetic fields and treat illness.	4
Biofeedback	A method of learning to control certain body functions voluntarily such as heartbeat, blood pressure, and muscle tension with the help of a special machine.	3

Term	Definition	Ref
	This method can help control pain.	1
Biofield therapy	Various forms of energy work to assist in healing.	4
Biological therapy	Treatments used to help the immune system fight disease in the body.	4
Biomarker	A measurable substance found in body fluid or tissue that may be a sign of disease or infection.	4
Biopsy	Process of removing tissue samples, which are then examined under a microscope to check for disease.	4
Biopsy specimen	Tissue removed from the body and examined under a microscope to determine whether disease is present.	4
Blog	A website that functions as an online diary or commentary on a particular subject. A blog may combine text, images, audio, video, and links to other online resources. Many blogs allow readers to leave comments or responses regarding the author's content. The term blog is a fusion of the words web and log (web log).	2
Blood Clot	A clump of blood that forms in a vein either just under the skin surface or in a deep vein. A blood clot that forms in a deep vein is called deep vein thrombosis, or DVT. See Deep Vein Thrombosis.	2
Blood vessel	A tube through which the blood circulates in the body. Blood vessels include a network of arteries, arterioles, capillaries, venules, and veins.	3
Body of the Pancreas	The middle part of the pancreas between the neck and the tail. The superior	1

Term	Definition	Ref
	mesenteric blood vessels run behind this part of the gland.	
Borderline resectable pancreatic cancer	Cancer that is confined to the pancreas but that approaches nearby structures or causes severe symptoms, so that it might not be possible to remove all the cancer with surgery.	4
Bowel	The small and large intestine.	4
BRCA1 and BRCA 2 genes	These are human genes that produce tumor suppressor proteins. These proteins help repair damaged DNA. Those who are positive for BRCA2 gene are at a higher risk for getting ovarian, breast, prostate or pancreatic cancer.	3
BRCA1 gene	A gene that normally helps to suppress cell growth; a person who inherits an altered version of this gene has a higher risk of getting breast, ovarian, or prostate cancer, and possibly pancreatic cancer.	4
BRCA2 gene	A gene that normally helps to suppress cell growth; a person who inherits an altered version of this gene has a higher risk of getting breast, ovarian, prostate, or pancreatic cancer.	4
Brush biopsy	A procedure used with endoscopic retrograde cholangiopancreatography (ERCP); a small brush is inserted through an endoscope and into the bile duct and pancreatic duct to scrape the inside of the ducts to collect cells for examination.	4
Bypass	A surgical procedure in which the doctor creates a new pathway for the flow of body fluids.	3

Term	Definition	Ref
CA19-9	A blood marker for pancreas cancer. It is not a good screening test for diagnosing possible pancreas cancers in individuals without symptoms. Instead, it can be useful in following the progress of patients known to have a cancer by measuring how their cancer is responding to treatment.	1
Cachexia	A condition causing weight loss and muscle wasting that occurs in advanced cancer, among other diseases.	4
Calories	Energy available in food.	2
Cancer	Any of a group of diseases in which the cells are abnormal, grow out of control, and can spread.	4
Cancer Cachexia (pronounced kə kéksee ə)	A cancer-related condition marked by weight loss due to the body's improper use of calories and proteins. Cancer cachexia creates fatigue and weakness and may impair the body's response to treatment.	2
Cancer screening	The use of tests to find cancer before signs of cancer appear.	4
Cancer stage	See Clinical stage, Staging cancer, and Stage.	4
Cancer stem cells	Subpopulation of cancer cells believed to be responsible for starting and maintaining the cancer.	4
Cancer-Fighting Treatment	Any cancer treatment whose goal is curative in nature. Cancer-fighting treatments may include surgery, chemotherapy, radiation therapy, targeted therapy, and/or immunotherapy. Once treatments to fight the cancer are no longer an option, survivors will only receive treatments that improve quality of life (See Palliative Care).	2

Term	Definition	Ref
Capecitabine (Xeloda)	One of the approved chemotherapy drugs for pancreatic cancer, it gets metabolized into 5-FU; in either form the drug disrupts the cell replication cycle.	4
Carbohydrate	A nutrient found in food. Carbohydrates are the preferred fuel for most body functions. With the exception of milk, foods high in carbohydrates are derived from plant sources.	2
Carcinoembryonic antigen (CEA)	A protein that may sometimes be found in the blood of people who have certain types of cancers, and not usually found in healthy persons.	4
Carcinogen	Cancer-causing agent.	4
Carcinoma	Cancer that starts in cells that form the lining of structures of the body.	4
Carcinoma in situ	Abnormal or cancer cells that have not grown into the next layer of tissue.	4
Care Plan	A strategy that is based on meeting the cancer survivor's individualized needs.	2
Caregiver	A term used to mean whoever is providing most of the survivor's day-to-day care, whether that person is a spouse, partner, parent, child, sibling, relative, or privately hired person. This person is also referred to as the primary caregiver.	2
Caregivers	Persons who provide help with daily activities, coordinate healthcare and other services, and provide emotional and other types of support for patients.	4
Catheter	A flexible tube used to deliver fluids into, or withdraw fluids out of, the body.	4

Term	Definition	Ref
Celiac artery	Supplies oxygenated blood to the stomach, liver, spleen, and parts of the esophagus, duodenum, and pancreas. Also known as the celiac axis.	4
Celiac Axis	A short, thick artery arising from the largest artery in the body, the aorta. The celiac axis starts just below the diaphragm and divides almost immediately into the gastric, hepatic, and splenic arteries.	2
Celiac plexus	Complex network of nerves in the abdomen.	4
Celiac plexus block	Injections of pain medications given to relieve abdominal pain, often used in cancer treatment or chronic pancreatitis. The pain is believed to be caused by irritation of the celiac plexus, a network of nerves surrounding the aorta.	4
Cell	The individual unit that makes up the tissues of the body. All living things are made up of one or more cells.	3
Chemo brain	A problem with thinking and memory that can happen during and especially after chemotherapy treatment for cancer. Also known as chemo fog.	4
Chemoradiation	Radiation therapy used in combination with chemotherapy.	4
Chemotherapy	Use of drugs to kill cancer cells.	4
Chemotherapy cycle	Days of treatment followed by days of rest.	4
Chemotherapy sensitivity testing	Pre-testing chemotherapies to determine which drugs are most effective against a cancer before undergoing a complete course of therapy.	4

Term	Definition	Ref
Chiropractic	A health profession concerned with the diagnosis, treatment, and prevention of mechanical disorders of the muscles and bones, and the effects of these disorders on the function of the nervous system and general health; it emphasizes manual treatments, including spinal manipulation.	4
Chronic pain	Pain that occurs over a long period of time that may range from mild to severe.	4
Chronic pancreatitis	Condition in which inflammation irreversibly damages the pancreas; or chronic damage with persistent pain or malabsorption.	4
Circulating tumor cells (CTCs)	Cells may shed from tumors and be found in small numbers in the bloodstream of certain cancer patients. These cells are known as circulating tumor cells (CTCs). CTCs are considered to be the source of cells that spread and form metastases in other organs.	4
Cisplatin	One of the approved chemotherapy drugs for pancreatic cancer, it is a platinum-based drug that disrupts DNA and kills cancer cells.	4
Clinical stage	The rating of the extent of cancer based on tests before treatment. (See also Stage and Staging cancer.)	4
Clinical trial	The study of a drug, procedure, or medical device to determine its safety and effectiveness in people; there are many types of clinical trials used to find better ways to prevent, screen for, diagnose, and treat disease, and to improve quality of life. (See also Phases of clinical trials.)	4

Term	Definition	Ref
Coexisting condition	Occurring at the same time but independent of another condition or illness.	4
Common bile duct	The tube in the body that carries bile from the liver and gallbladder into the duodenum (the upper part of the small intestine).	3
Complementary therapy	Treatment methods added to conventional or traditional therapy.	4
Computed Tomography Scan (CT scan)	A series of detailed pictures of areas inside the body taken from different angles. The pictures are created by a computer linked to an x-ray machine.	3
Constipation	A condition of the digestive system in which a person experiences hard stools that are difficult to eliminate; constipation may be painful and, in severe cases, may lead to a blockage of the bowel.	4
Contraindicate	to state something to be inadvisable while taking certain medication because of a likely adverse reaction.	3
Contrast agent (or medium)	A dye, taken by mouth or injected, that is sometimes used during x-ray examinations to highlight areas that otherwise might not be seen.	1
Contrast material	A dye or other substance that helps show abnormal areas inside the body. It is given by injection into a vein, by enema, or by mouth. Contrast material may be used with x-rays, CT scans, MRI, or other imaging tests.	3
Coping	How people or family members come to terms with an illness, make decisions, solve problems, and adapt to life's changes, while still feeling good about themselves.	4

Term	Definition	Ref
Curative treatment	Treatment used to fully rid the body of a disease.	4
Cyst	A sac or capsule in the body. It is usually filled with fluid or other material.	3
Cytokines	A group of compounds that allow cells to communicate with each other. During normal functioning, cytokines help the immune system respond quickly. In pancreatic cancer, cytokines can influence the rate at which nutrients are metabolized.	2
Cytology	A branch of biology dealing with the structure, function, multiplication, pathology, and life history of cells.	3
Data Safety Monitoring Board (DSMB)	An impartial group that oversees an ongoing clinical trial and reviews the results to determine if they are acceptable. This group determines if the trial should be modified or closed at any time during the trial.	2
Debulking surgery	Surgery that removes as much of the cancer as possible.	4
Deep margin	Normal-looking tissue beneath a tumor.	4
Deep margin status	The presence or absence of cancer cells in the normal-looking tissue under a tumor that is removed by surgery.	4
Deep Vein Thrombosis (DVT)	The formation of a blood clot in a deep vein, generally in the lower extremities. DVT can cause serious problems if it breaks loose and travels through the bloodstream to the lung. Symptoms of DVT include swelling, pain when walking or flexing the foot and sometimes redness in one leg.	2
Deoxyribonucleic	The molecules inside cells that carry genetic information and pass it from one generation	2

Term	Definition	Ref
Acid (DNA)	to the next.	
Diabetes mellitus	Disease in which the body does not properly control the amount of sugar in the blood, resulting in high levels; it occurs when the body does not produce enough or any insulin or does not use it properly.	4
Diaphragm	A dome shaped muscle that separates the lungs and heart from the abdomen. This muscle assists in breathing.	1
Diarrhea	A condition marked by frequent and loose bowel movements.	2
Dietitian	A dietitian is a healthcare professional trained in food, nutrition, biochemistry and physiology. A dietitian can provide guidance regarding an appropriate diet for the patient with pancreatic cancer.	2
Distal pancreatectomy	Surgical procedure in which the tail and body of the pancreas are removed, usually along with the entire spleen; sometimes, part of the body of the pancreas can be preserved.	4
Diuretic	A substance that promotes increased urine excretion.	2
DNA (deoxyribonucleic acid)	The molecule in the cell nucleus that carries the instructions for making living organisms.	4
Dosage	A determined amount of a prescribed drug.	2
Drug interaction	A change in the way a drug acts or works in the body when it is taken with another drug or substance; the interaction can cause unwanted effects.	4

Term	Definition	Ref
Drug resistance	When a formerly effective medication stops being effective against a disease.	4
Dual-phase helical CT scan	Imaging test for evaluating patients suspected of having pancreatic cancer; this type of computed tomography scan can detect about 98 percent of pancreatic cancers.	4
Duct	A channel leading from an exocrine gland or organ.	4
Dumping	A condition in which there is rapid emptying of the stomach shortly after eating. It may be characterized by flushed skin, weakness, dizziness, abdominal pain, nausea, vomiting and/or diarrhea.	2
Duodenum	The first part of the small intestine that connects to the stomach.	4
Durable power of attorney for healthcare	The legal designation of a person responsible to make medical decisions for a patient when that patient cannot do so.	4
Early-stage cancer	Cancer that has had little or no growth into nearby tissues.	4
Eastern Cooperative Oncology Group (ECOG) Performance Scale	A rating scale of one's ability to do daily activities.	4
-ectomy	Surgical removal of a structure or part of a structure. For example, pancreatectomy is the surgical removal of the pancreas (or a portion of it).	1
Edema	Swelling around tissue due to the buildup of fluid.	4

Term	Definition	Ref
Efficacy	Effectiveness: the power to produce a desired result.	4
Electrolytes	Electrically charged minerals that help to maintain (1) the proper amount and kind of fluid in every compartment of the body, and (2) the acid-base (pH) balance of the body. Electrolytes include sodium, potassium, chloride, and magnesium.	2
Eligibility Requirements	A set of basic qualifying standards that must be met in order to participate in a clinical trial. Participants are selected by these inclusion and exclusion criteria.	2
Endocrine	Refers to tissue that makes and releases hormones that travel in the bloodstream and control the actions of other cells or organs. Some examples of endocrine tissues are the pancreas, pituitary, thyroid, and adrenal glands.	3
Endocrine gland	A gland that secretes its hormone directly into the bloodstream that flows through it, rather than through an opening; endocrine tissue comprises 5 percent of the pancreas.	4
Endocrinologist	A physician who specializes in disorders of glands of the endocrine system.	4
Endoscope	Thin, tube-like instrument used to look at tissue inside the body; an endoscope has a light and a lens for viewing and may have a tool to remove tissue.	4
Endoscopic biopsy	A type of biopsy that uses a long, thin tube with a camera on the end to go down the esophagus to remove tissue samples.	4
Endoscopic retrograde cholangiopancreatog	Minimally invasive procedure during which a thin, lighted tube is passed down the throat, through the stomach and small	4

Term	Definition	Ref
raphy (ERCP)	intestine, and into the bile duct and pancreatic duct to view them for obstruction and to take X-rays.	
Endoscopic UItrasound (EUS)	A procedure in which an endoscope is inserted into the body. An endoscope is a thin, tube-like instrument that has a light and a lens for viewing. A probe at the end of the endoscope is used to bounce high-energy sound waves (ultrasound) off internal organs to make a picture (sonogram).	3
Enzymes	Proteins that speed up chemical reactions in the body and that the body produces naturally; enzymes help the body with functions such as digesting food.	4
Epidermal growth factor receptor (EGFR)	A protein on the edge of a cell that sends signals for the cell to grow.	4
Erlotinib hydrochloride (Tarceva)	One of the approved chemotherapy drugs for pancreatic cancer, it is a receptor kinase inhibitor and prevents cancer cells from multiplying.	4
Esophagus	The tube that connects the throat with the stomach; the esophagus lies between the trachea (windpipe) and the spine; it passes down the neck, pierces the diaphragm, and joins the upper end of the stomach.	4
Everolimus (Afinitor®)	A targeted therapy drug approved in 2011 by the FDA to treat advanced pancreatic neuroendocrine tumors. It inhibits the growth of cancer cells by blocking the Mammalian Target of Rapamycin (mTOR) protein. It may also stop the formation of blood vessels that provide nutrients and oxygen to the tumor.	2

Term	Definition	Ref
Excision	Removal by surgery.	4
Excisional biopsy	Removal of an entire tumor to test for disease.	4
Exclusion Criteria	A set of standards used to determine participants who are not eligible to participate in a clinical trial.	2
Exocrine	Refers to tissue that makes and releases substances into a duct (tube). Some ducts lead to other organs but most lead out of the body. Some examples of exocrine tissues are the tear glands, sweat glands, and the pancreas.	3
Exocrine gland	A gland that secretes its fluid through a duct; exocrine tissue comprises 95 percent of the pancreas.	4
Experimental Treatment	A drug, medical device, or a combination of treatments being tested in humans for use in a specific disease or disorder. An experimental treatment for pancreatic cancer may or may not already have FDA approval to treat another disease or condition. Also called an investigational treatment/therapy.	2
External beam radiation therapy	Treatment for cancer in which a beam of high-dose radiation is focused on the tumor from outside of the body.	4
Familial	A trait that is common within a family who is genetically related. These traits are inherited through genes passed from one generation to the next.	2
Familial atypical multiple mole melanoma	Genetic syndrome in which many different-sized, asymmetrical, raised moles are present; may be associated with melanoma	4

Term	Definition	Ref
(FAMMM) syndrome	or pancreatic cancer.	
Familial breast cancer syndrome	Breast cancer that occurs more often in a family than would normally occur by chance. There is often a genetic factor, such as a BRCA mutation, which increases the risk of several cancers, including pancreatic cancer.	4
Familial pancreatic cancer	Pancreatic cancer that occurs more often in a family than would normally occur by chance. There is often a genetic factor (known or unknown) involved.	4
FDR	First Degree relatives - Blood relatives in your immediate family: parents, children, and siblings	1
Fine-needle aspiration (FNA) biopsy	Technique in which a thin needle is inserted into a tumor; cells are removed and examined under a microscope.	4
First Line Therapy	The first type of treatment given for a condition or disease.	2
First-degree relative	Parents, children, or siblings of an individual.	4
First-line treatment	The first set of treatments given to treat a disease.	4
Fluorouracil (also knowns as 5-FU and 5-fluorouracil)	A chemotherapy drug used to treat pancreatic cancer. It is also used as part of the combination of drugs known as FOLFIRINOX.	4
FOLFIRINOX	One of the standard treatments for advanced pancreatic cancer. It is a four-drug combination: FOL (leucovorin calcium, or folinic acid), F (fluorouracil, or 5-FU), IRIN (irinotecan), OX (oxaliplatin). Each of these	4

Term	Definition	Ref
	drugs enhances the action of the others.	
FOLFOX	A combination chemotherapy consisting of leucovorin (folinic acid), fluorouracil, and oxaliplatin.	4
Follow-up testing	Tests done after treatment to check for signs that the cancer has come back.	4
Food and Drug Administration (FDA)	A federal agency that promotes and protects public health by ensuring the safety and effectiveness of medical treatments.	2
Four-dimensional computed tomography (4D-CT)	A CT scan that can show the movement of organs.	4
Gallbladder	Pear-shaped organ located under the liver in which bile is concentrated and stored.	4
Gallstone	A solid build-up that forms in the common bile duct or the gallbladder. Gallstones are usually made of cholesterol and other substances found in the gallbladder. One large stone or many little ones may form.	2
Gastrin	The major hormone that regulates acid secretion in the stomach.	2
Gastroenterologist	A physician who specializes in disorders of the digestive system.	4
Gastrointestinal (GI) tract	The group of organs through which food passes after being eaten.	4
Gemcitabine (Gemzar®)	A chemotherapy drug approved by the U.S. FDA in 1996 as the standard of care treatment for pancreatic cancer.	2
Gene	The functional and physical unit of heredity passed from parent to child; most genes contain the information for making a	4

Term	Definition	Ref
	specific protein. Genes are composed of DNA.	
General anesthesia	A temporary loss of feeling and a complete loss of awareness that feels like a very deep sleep. It is caused by special drugs or other substances called anesthetics. General anesthesia keeps patients from feeling pain during surgery or other procedures.	3
Genetic	Having to do with genes and the information in genes.	4
Genetic counseling	Discussion with a counselor with specific expertise in diseases caused by abnormal cells that are inherited from family members.	4
Genetic Counselor	A health professional with a graduate degree in medical genetics and counseling. Genetic counselors work with families who may be at risk for a variety of inherited conditions. They help families identify and understand inherited diseases and help them interpret how that information applies to their individual situation.	2
Genetic mutation	A change in the DNA sequence that makes a gene different from what is normally seen. Mutations cause many different variances in genes, and the majority are harmless. But some mutations make people more likely to develop certain diseases, including cancer.	4
Genetic risk	The chance of getting a disease due to gene mutations that are inherited.	4
Genetic testing	Medical testing of a person's DNA, which can identify changes in chromosomes, genes, or proteins that indicate the existence of a genetic disorder or disease.	4

Term	Definition	Ref
Genome	The full set of genes of an organism.	4
Germline mutation	A change in the genes of the sperm or egg cells, which becomes part of the DNA of any offspring. Also called hereditary mutation.	4
Gland	An organ that makes one or more substances, such as hormones, digestive juices, sweat, tears, saliva, or milk. Endocrine glands release the substances directly into the bloodstream. Exocrine glands release the substances into a duct or opening to the inside or outside of the body.	3
Glucagon	a hormone produced by the pancreas that raises the blood sugar level by promoting the conversion of glycogen to glucose in the liver.	3
Glucose	A simple sugar that provides a major energy source for the body. Carbohydrates are metabolized to form glucose for use by the body.	2
Glucose Intolerance	A condition marked by elevated blood glucose levels. Symptoms include high thirst, frequent urination, and fatigue.	2
GVAX pancreas vaccine	An experimental immunotherapy that stimulates different aspects of the immune system to kill tumor cells.	4
Head of the pancreas	The widest part of the pancreas. It is found in the right part of the abdomen, nestled in the curve of the duodenum.	4
Health care proxy	A person chosen by the patient to make medical decisions for that patient.	4
Helical ("Spiral") CT	A diagnostic technique which provides information about the nature and site of the	3

Term	Definition	Ref
scan	lesion (e.g., pancreatic vs. other periampullary tumors, bile duct tumors), its resectability (e.g., liver metastases, vascular invasion), and vascular anatomy.	
Hepatic	Relating to or affecting the liver.	3
Hepatic artery	A short blood vessel branching off the celiac artery. It brings oxygenated blood to the liver, pylorus of the stomach, pancreas, and duodenum.	4
Hepatitis	Inflammation of the liver.	4
Hereditary	A trait that is carried by genes from one generation to the next.	2
Hereditary cancer	Cancer that is caused by a genetic abnormality that was passed from parent to child.	4
Hereditary nonpolyposis colon cancer (HNPCC; Lynch syndrome)	Syndrome in which there is a higher-than-normal chance of developing colon, pancreatic, uterine, stomach, or ovarian cancer.	4
Hereditary pancreatitis	Rare disease in which patients develop episodes of recurrent pancreatitis at an early age.	4
Home Care	The most common type of hospice in which the hospice staff visits the private home to assess the survivor's condition and manage symptoms. Most of the survivor's day-to-day care is provided by a family member or close friend.	2
Homeopathic medicine	System of medicine based on the premise that "like cures like"; practitioners believe that a substance that produces a set of symptoms in a healthy person will, in small doses, cure those symptoms in a person	4

Term	Definition	Ref
	with a disease.	
Hormone	One of many chemicals made by glands in the body. Hormones circulate in the bloodstream and control the actions of certain cells or organs. Some hormones can also be made in the laboratory.	3
Hospice	Concept of care that emphasizes palliative care rather than cures, quality of life over quantity, and comfort measures for patients provided at home, at a hospice facility, or in a hospital.	4
Hospice Team	A group of health professionals who work with the caregivers to provide end-of-life care for the cancer survivor. The health professionals on the hospice team include the hospice physician, hospice registered nurse, home health aides/certified nursing assistants, social worker, chaplain, volunteers, and bereavement counselor.	2
Hypnosis	A trance-like state in which a person becomes more aware and focused and is more open to suggestion.	3
Ileum	Lowest part of the small intestine, located beyond the duodenum and jejunum, just before the large intestine (the colon).	4
Image-guided radiation therapy (IGRT)	Treatment with radiation that uses imaging tests to better target the tumor.	4
Imagery	Technique in which people focus on positive images in their mind.	3
Imaging tests	Methods used to produce pictures of internal body structures; for example, X-ray films, ultrasonography, computed tomography (CT) scans, and magnetic	4

Term	Definition	Ref
	resonance imaging (MRI).	
Immune cells	Cells that are part of the body's natural defense against infection and disease.	4
Immune response	The action of the body's natural defense against infection and disease in response to a foreign substance.	4
Immune suppression	The condition in which the body's immune system, its natural defense against infection and disease, is weakened. This can occur because of illness or because of treatment for some diseases.	4
Immune system	The body's natural defense against disease, made up of a variety of organs, cells, and proteins.	4
Immunoglobulin	Proteins in the serum and cells of the immune system that help fight off infection. Also called antibodies.	4
Immunohistochemistry (IHC)	A test of proteins within cells to detect specific cell traits involved in abnormal cell growth. It is used to diagnose types of cancer.	4
Immunotherapy	Treatment that boosts the body's natural defense against disease. Also called immune therapy.	4
In situ	Literally, something found in its original place. In cancer in situ describes cancer cells that have not spread from their original location.	4
Incidental finding	During evaluation for a disease, finding another disease unintentionally.	4
Incision	A cut made in the body to perform surgery.	3

Term	Definition	Ref
Incisional biopsy	Surgery that removes a tissue sample from a tumor to test for cancer cells.	4
Inclusion Criteria	A set of standards used to select participants who are eligible to participate in a clinical trial.	2
Inflammation	A reaction in one part of the body that produces redness, warmth, swelling, and pain as a result of infection, irritation, or injury. Inflammation can be external or internal.	4
Informed consent	Process in which a person is given important facts, such as the risks and benefits, about a medical procedure or treatment or a clinical trial before deciding whether to participate.	4
Informed consent form	A document that must be read, understood, and signed by a person wanting to take part in a research study or clinical trial.	4
Infusion	A method of giving drugs slowly through a needle into a vein.	4
Inherited mutations	DNA mutations carried in a person's reproductive cells and potentially passed on to that person's children. (see also Mutations.)	4
Inpatient Hospice Care	A type of hospice care that is delivered in healthcare facilities, such as a hospice facility, hospital, or nursing home. It is used when pain and other symptoms cannot be addressed at home.	2
Insoluble Fiber	A tough, indigestible fiber that does not dissolve readily in water. Food sources include fruits, vegetables, seeds, nuts, legumes, and whole grains. Possible health effects include softened stools, regulation of	2

Term	Definition	Ref
	bowel movements, and lowered blood cholesterol.	
Institutional Review Board (IRB)	A group of scientists, doctors, clergy, advocates, and consumers at each health care facility that protects the participants by reviewing and approving the action plan for every clinical trial. The IRB checks to see that the trial is well-designed and does not involve unreasonable risks.	2
Insulin	A hormone made by islet cells of the pancreas that controls the amount of sugar in the blood by moving it into the cells, where it can be used for energy.	4
Integrative Medicine	A type of medical care that combines conventional (standard) medical treatment with complementary and alternative (CAM) therapies that have been shown to be safe and to work. CAM therapies treat the mind, body, and spirit.	3
Integrative therapy	Combined use of a proven treatment and a complementary therapy.	4
Interstitial radiation	A type of internal radiation therapy that places radioactive objects in the tumor.	4
Interventional radiologist	A radiologist who uses image guidance methods to gain access to vessels and organs to treat diseases.	4
Intestine	The long, tube-shaped organ in the abdomen that completes the process of digestion. The intestine has two parts, the small intestine, and the large intestine. Also called bowel.	3
Intraductal papillary mucinous neoplasm	A tumor of the pancreas that produces mucus that clogs and enlarges the pancreatic duct; IPMNs may progress to invasive	4

Term	Definition	Ref
(IPMN)	pancreatic cancer if left untreated.	
Intraoperative	During the course of surgery.	4
Intraoperative radiation therapy (IORT)	Radiation therapy given during surgery.	4
Intraperitoneal (IP) chemotherapy	Drugs given by a small tube surgically placed in the abdomen.	4
Intrathecal injection	Injection into the space surrounding the spinal cord.	4
Intravenous	Into or within a vein. Intravenous usually refers to a way of giving a drug or other substance through a needle or tube inserted into a vein. Also called IV.	3
Intravenous (IV) chemotherapy	Drugs given by a needle or tube inserted into a vein.	4
Intravenous injection	Injection directly into a vein.	4
Irinotecan	One of the approved chemotherapy drugs for pancreatic cancer, it inhibits the replication and transcription of DNA, and so interferes with cell growth.	4
Islet cell	A pancreatic cell that produces hormones (such as insulin and glucagon) that are secreted into the bloodstream. These hormones help control the level of glucose (sugar) in the blood. Also called endocrine pancreas cell and islet of Langerhans cell.	3
Islet cell tumor	A tumor that arises from the islet cells of the pancreas, which may be benign or cancerous.	4
Islets of Langerhans	Collections of cells in the pancreas that produce insulin and glucagon, important	4

Term	Definition	Ref
	regulators of sugar metabolism.	
Jaundice	Condition in which the skin and the whites of the eyes become yellow, urine may become dark, and stool may become clay-colored; occurs when the liver is not working properly, or a bile duct is blocked.	4
Jejunostomy	A surgical operation that creates access from the outside of the body into the middle part of the small intestine so that nourishment can be directly introduced.	3
Jejunostomy Tube (j-tube)	A feeding tube inserted through the abdomen into the small intestine, bypassing the stomach. Special liquid food is given to the patient through the j-tube. Pancreatic enzymes may be added to the liquid to aid in the breakdown and absorption of nutrients.	2
Jejunum	Portion of the small intestine that extends from the duodenum to the ileum.	4
Karnofsky Performance Status Scale (KPS)	A rating scale of one's ability to do daily activities.	4
Karyotype	A map of chromosomes according to their size and shape. Karyotyping is a process that examines a map (karyotype) of a cell's chromosomes.	4
KRAS gene	A gene capable of causing cancer when altered; drugs that block its activity may stop cancer growth. Sometimes called K-ras oncogene.	4
Lactase	The enzyme necessary to break down the sugar lactose.	2
Lactose	The natural sugar found in milk and milk	2

Term	Definition	Ref
	products.	
Lactose Intolerance	A condition in which the body's digestive system is unable to completely metabolize lactose. It is often caused by insufficient amounts of lactase.	2
Lanreotide acetate (Somatuline Depot)	One of the approved drugs for treating symptoms of pancreatic neuroendocrine tumors.	4
Laparoscope	Small telescope-like instrument connected to a video monitor.	4
Laparoscopic ultrasonography	Procedure that uses a laparoscope, inserted through the abdominal wall, and is guided by ultrasonography.	4
Laparoscopy	Procedure during which a laparoscope is inserted through a small incision in the abdomen by which the internal organs can be viewed, and tissue samples removed for examination.	4
Leucovorin calcium	A drug derived from folic acid that improves how well 5-FU, a type of chemotherapy, works.	4
Lipase	An enzyme secreted by the pancreas that breaks down fats.	2
Liquid biopsy	Tests on blood samples that look for pieces of tumor or tumor DNA circulating in the blood.	4
Liver	The largest solid organ in the body, situated in the upper part of the abdomen on the right side, the liver filters toxins out of the blood and synthesizes a number of important proteins and biochemicals.	4

Term	Definition	Ref
Living will	One of several documents called advance directives that designate what kind of medical care a patient wants, or does not want, in the event the patient cannot speak for himself or herself.	4
Local anesthesia	Drugs given to cause a loss of feeling in a small area of the body.	4
Locally advanced	Cancer that is confined to the area around affected organ but cannot be surgically removed because the tumor may be intertwined with major blood vessels and may have invaded surrounding organs. There is no evidence of spread to other areas of the body.	4
Loco-regional pancreatic cancer	A primary pancreatic cancer that has spread to regional lymph nodes and/or resectable (removable) tissues. Removable tissues include some lymph nodes and parts of the duodenum and stomach that are routinely removed in some surgical treatments for pancreatic cancer.	1
Long-term side effect	A negative physical response to treatment that continues for months or years after finishing treatment.	4
Low-dose computed tomography (LDCT)	A test that uses little amounts of radiation to make pictures of the inside of the body.	4
Low-dose rate brachytherapy	Treatment with radioactive objects that are inserted into a tumor and left to decay.	4
Lutathera (lutetium Lu 177 dotatate)	One of the approved chemotherapy drugs for pancreatic cancer, this radioactive drug binds to a cell receptor and enters the cell, allowing radiation to cause damage to the tumor cells.	4

Term	Definition	Ref
Lymph node	A rounded mass of lymphatic tissue that is surrounded by a capsule of connective tissue. Lymph nodes filter lymph (lymphatic fluid), and they store lymphocytes (white blood cells). They are located along lymphatic vessels. Also called lymph gland.	3
Lymph nodes	Small, bean-shaped structures in the neck, underarm, groin, chest, abdomen, pelvis, near the pancreas, and throughout the body; they store white blood cells.	4
Lymph System	The tissues and organs that produce, store, and carry white blood cells that filter and fight infections and other diseases. This system includes the bone marrow, spleen, thymus, lymph nodes, and lymphatic vessels.	2
Lymph vessel	A thin tube that carries lymph (lymphatic fluid) and white blood cells through the lymphatic system. Also called lymphatic vessel.	3
Lymphatic fluid	Fluid that circulates through the lymph vessels and empties into blood vessels in the upper chest.	4
Lymphatic system	The body's complex set of lymph nodes, lymph cells, and lymph vessels that fight infection and disease.	4
Lymphocyte	A type of white blood cell that helps fight infection and disease.	4
Magnetic resonance cholangiopancreatog raphy (MRCP)	Imaging method that is safe and fast; a form of magnetic resonance imaging (MRI) used to view the bile duct and pancreatic duct.	4
Magnetic resonance imaging (MRI)	Imaging method that uses powerful magnets to view internal organs and structures; the energy from the magnets is absorbed by the	4

Term	Definition	Ref
	body and released. A computer translates the energy patterns into detailed images of areas inside the body.	
Magnetic resonance spectroscopy	A test that measures chemicals in cells without removing tissue from the body.	4
Main pancreatic duct	A tube-shaped vessel that drains digestive fluids from the pancreas into the gut.	4
Maintenance treatment	Treatment given to help sustain good treatment results.	4
Malignant	Cancerous; malignant tumors can invade and destroy nearby tissues and spread to other parts of the body.	4
Malignant tumor	A cancer that has the potential of invading nearby tissues, spreading to other organs (metastasizing) and possibly leading to the patient's death.	1
Margins	Margins indicate the border or edge of the tissue removed during cancer surgery. The margins are said to be clear or negative when there are no cancer cells at the edge of the tissue, indicating that all the cancer has been removed.	3
MCT (Medium Chain Triglyceride) Oil	An easily absorbed form of fat added to medical nutritional products to increase caloric intake.	2
Medical oncologist	A physician who is trained to prescribe anticancer medications.	4
Melanoma	Serious form of skin cancer that begins in melanocytes (cells that make the pigment melanin).	4
Mesentery	A membrane that supports an organ or body part, especially the double-layered	3

Term	Definition	Ref
	membrane of the peritoneum attached to the back wall of the abdominal cavity that supports the small intestine.	
Metabolism (Metabolic)	All the chemical reactions occurring in the body that are necessary to maintain life. The human body metabolizes, or breaks down and rebuilds, nutrients from food for use within the cells.	2
Metastasis (Metastasize)	The spread of cancer from one part of the body to a distant organ.	2
Metastatic	Cancer that has spread beyond the area of the affected organ or part of the body and involves other organs, such as the liver or lungs, or other areas.	4
Metastatic cancer	A cancer that has spread from one organ to another. Pancreas cancer most frequently metastasizes to the liver. In general, cancers that have metastasized are generally not treated surgically, but instead are treated with chemotherapy and/or radiation therapy.	1
Microsatellitosis	Tiny tumors near the main tumor that can only be seen with a microscope.	4
Microscopic metastases	Cancer cells that have spread from the first tumor and cannot be seen by the naked eye.	4
Minimal residual disease (MRD)	A very small number of cancer cells left in the body after treatment that can't be seen with a microscope.	4
Minimally invasive surgery	The use of small tools inserted through small incisions to do surgery.	4
Mitomycin C	One of the approved chemotherapy drugs for pancreatic cancer, it works by sticking the cancer cell's DNA (the cell's genetic	4

Term	Definition	Ref
	code) together so that it can't come apart again. The cell can't divide so the cancer cannot grow.	
Modified Whipple procedure	Same as the Whipple procedure, except none of the stomach is removed. Also called Pylorus-preserving Whipple procedure.	3
Monitoring tests	Tests done during treatment to check if treatment is working.	4
Monoclonal antibody	A type of immune system protein made in a lab that can attach to substances in the body such as cancer cells.	4
Morbidity	The incidence of disease.	3
Multiagent chemotherapy	The use of two or more cancer drugs in one treatment, to get a stronger effect against the disease.	4
Multidetector row helical CT (MDCT) Scan	Helical CT scanner with multiple detector rows; advantages over other CT scanners include improved image resolution and rapid scanning of large volumes.	4
Multidisciplinary care	Team approach to the care of patients with cancer in which physicians in many different areas of specialization join to provide their expertise and experience.	4
Multiple endocrine neoplasia type 1 syndrome (MEN1; Wermer's syndrome)	A rare, inherited disorder that affects the endocrine glands and can cause tumors in the pancreas and other organs, which usually are not cancerous.	4
Mutation	A change in the DNA of a cell. Certain mutations can lead to cancer. Mutations can be inherited or can occur over the course of a lifetime.	2

Term	Definition	Ref
Mutations	Errors in the DNA code that occur in the process of cell replication and division; certain mutations may lead to cancer or other diseases. (See also Inherited Mutations.)	4
Myocardial infarction	The death of a segment of heart muscle, caused by a blood clot in the coronary artery interrupting blood supply.	3
Nab-paclitaxel (Abraxane)	One of the approved chemotherapy drugs for pancreatic cancer, it inhibits cell division and promotes cell death. It is often given with gemcitabine.	4
Naturopathic medicine	Practitioners work with patients to provide nutritional and lifestyle counseling using dietary supplements, medicinal plants, and traditional Chinese medicine.	4
Nausea	A feeling of sickness in the stomach that prompts the urge to vomit.	2
Neck of the Pancreas	The thin section of the pancreas between the head and the body of the gland.	1
NED	No evidence of disease.	4
Needle biopsy	The removal of tissue or fluid with a needle for examination under a microscope. When a thick needle is used, the procedure is called a core biopsy. When a thin needle is used, the procedure is called a fine-needle aspiration biopsy.	3
Neoadjuvant chemo and radiation therapy	Chemotherapy and radiation therapy that is given to patients before surgery. Some centers feel that the use of neoadjuvant therapy improves local and regional control of disease and that it may make more patients surgical candidates.	1

Term	Definition	Ref
Neoplasm	New growth; a tumor that may be benign or malignant.	4
Nerve block	Procedure in which a local anesthetic is injected around a nerve to produce numbness or pain reduction.	4
Neuroablation	Cutting or destroying part of pain fibers to help control pain.	4
Neuroendocrine	Having to do with the interactions between the nervous system and the endocrine system.	4
Neuropathy	A nerve problem that causes pain, tingling, and numbness in the hands and feet.	4
Neutropenia	A disorder caused by low levels of neutrophils, a type of white blood cell.	4
Nodule	A small mass of tissue.	4
Nonmetastatic recurrence	Cancer that has come back after treatment but has not spread to parts of the body far away from the first (primary) tumor.	4
Nonsteroidal anti-inflammatory drugs (NSAIDs)	Drugs that reduce inflammation and pain.	4
Nurse Case Manager (Nurse Navigator)	A registered nurse who has special training in how to plan, manage, and evaluate all aspects of patient care, especially for patients who get treatment over a long time. Also called case management nurse.	3
Obese	The state of having too much body fat. Adults with a body max index of 30 or over are considered obese.	2
Obesity	A condition marked by an abnormally high, unhealthy amount of body fat.	3

Term	Definition	Ref
Oncologist	A physician who specializes in the diagnosis and treatment of cancer.	4
Oncology	A branch of medicine that treats cancer.	4
Oncology Nurses	Nurses with specialized training in managing the treatment and care of patients with cancer; they may administer chemotherapy drugs, help in management of side effects, and provide patient education.	4
Oncology Social Workers	Social workers professionally trained to counsel patients with cancer and help provide practical assistance, for example, by helping patients find support groups and locate services.	4
Oncology surgeons	A doctor who is an expert in cancer surgery.	4
Onivyde (irinotecan hydrochloride liposome)	One of the approved chemotherapy drugs for pancreatic cancer, this form of irinotecan is enclosed in a lipid sphere to extend the time the drug remains in the body, thus increasing treatment effect.	4
Onset	In medicine, the first appearance of the signs or symptoms of an illness.	4
Opioids	Strongest pain relievers available.	4
Organ	A part of the body that performs a specific function. For example, the heart is an organ.	3
Organoid	Tiny three-dimensional biological replica of a patient's pancreatic tumor, cultured in the lab to allow researchers to test treatments to see what might work best for that patient.	4
Osteopathic	Form of conventional medicine that emphasizes diseases arising in the musculoskeletal system.	4

Term	Definition	Ref
-ostomy	A surgically created opening in an organ that can also be referred to as an anastomosis. Sometimes when surgeons remove a segment of bowel, they create an ostomy to allow for the bowel contents to exit the body.	1
Oxaliplatin	One of the approved chemotherapy drugs for pancreatic cancer, it is a platinum compound that disrupts DNA and kills cancer cells.	4
Paclitaxel (Abraxane)	One of the approved chemotherapy drugs for pancreatic cancer, it inhibits cell division and promotes cell death. It is often given with gemcitabine. (See also Nab-paclitaxel.)	4
Pain Management Specialist	is a branch of medicine employing an interdisciplinary approach for easing the suffering and improving the quality of life of those living with pain.	3
Palliative	Any treatment that reduces the severity of a disease or its symptoms. Palliative care is often a part of the treatment plan for patients with advanced pancreatic cancer.	1
Palliative care	Healthcare that specializes in the relief of suffering and improvement in quality of life.	4
Palliative surgery	Any noncurative surgical procedure that may be used in patients with pancreatic cancer to help relieve symptoms such as jaundice, nausea, vomiting, and pain to improve quality of life.	4
Pancreas	An organ of the digestive system located deep in the abdomen that produces both pancreatic enzymes to aid in the digestion of food and hormones such as insulin.	4

Term	Definition	Ref
Pancreatectomy	A surgical procedure in which part or all of the pancreas is removed.	4
Pancreatic	Having to do with the pancreas.	3
Pancreatic cancer	A malignant tumor of the pancreas. There are two main types: adenocarcinoma, which makes up the vast majority of cases, and neuroendocrine cancer, which is the remaining 5 percent of cases.	4
Pancreatic cyst	Saclike pouches of fluid within the pancreas. Most do not cause symptoms and are not cancerous, but some can become malignant.	4
Pancreatic duct	Main duct that runs along the entire length of the pancreas and merges with the bile duct.	4
Pancreatic enzymes	Proteins produced by the pancreas to aid in the digestion of food.	4
Pancreatic intraepithelial neoplasia (PanIN)	Lesions too small to see with the naked eye that can progress to invasive pancreatic cancer over time.	4
Pancreatic juice	Fluid made by the pancreas. Pancreatic juices contain proteins called enzymes that aid in digestion.	3
Pancreatic neuroendocrine tumor (PNET)	This type of pancreatic tumor develops from the abnormal growth of endocrine (hormone-producing) cells in the pancreas called islet cells. PNETs grow more slowly and may have a higher survival rate. Not all types of PNETs are cancerous.	4
Pancreaticoduodenectomy	Surgical procedure in patients with pancreatic cancer that removes part of the stomach, the duodenum, the head of the pancreas, part of the bile duct, the gallbladder, and lymph nodes in the area of	4

Term	Definition	Ref
	the pancreas (See Whipple procedure.)	
Pancreatitis	Inflammation of the pancreas.	4
Pancreatoduodenect omy	Removal of the head of the pancreas and parts of other nearby organs. Also called a Whipple procedure.	4
Papillary	A descriptive term that refers to a finger-like projection.	2
Paracentesis	A surgical procedure to remove fluid from the abdomen.	2
Pathologist	A physician trained to examine cells under a microscope for the diagnosis of cancer and other diseases.	4
Pathology report	A document with information about cells and tissue removed from the body and examined with a microscope for disease.	4
Patient-controlled analgesia (PCA)	Method of pain relief, commonly used after surgery in the immediate postoperative period, in which the patient controls the amount of pain medication by pressing a button on a computerized pump connected to a small tube in the body; patients cannot use more than the prescribed amount because the device is programmed for a maximum dosage.	4
Peri-ampullary	Around the ampulla of Vater in the duodenum. The peri-ampullary region is comprised of 4 structures: the ampulla, the duodenum, the bile duct and the head of the pancreas. It is sometimes difficult to tell which structure a tumor originated in. In such cases the diagnosis will be a peri-ampullary tumor.	1

Term	Definition	Ref
Peritoneum	Membrane that lines the abdominal cavity and covers most of the abdominal organs.	4
Personal Care	A type of caregiving that involves assisting the cancer survivor with activities of daily living including eating, dressing, bathing, grooming, using the toilet, and other needs. Providing personal care is often the most physically and emotionally challenging aspect of caregiving.	2
Peutz-Jeghers syndrome (PJS)	Genetic disorder in which polyps form in the intestine and dark spots appear on the mouth and fingers, and that increases the risk of developing many types of cancer, including pancreatic cancer.	4
Pharmacist	A person licensed to prepare and dispense (give out) prescription drugs and who has been taught how they work, how to use them, and their side effects.	3
Phase	A step in the course of the clinical trials process. There are four phases of clinical trials.	2
Phases of clinical trials	Sequential steps of clinical trials designed to answer specific questions and build on information from the previous phase. Phase 1: Determines the side effects of a new drug by gradually increasing the dosage and analyzing patients' responses. Phase 2: Determines if the new drug has the potential to be better than current treatments. Phase 3: Determines if the treatment is better than, as good as, or not as good as the accepted standard treatment. Phase 4: Examine long-term effective-ness and ad-verse effects after FDA approval.	4
Photon beam	Uses X-ray beams to get to the tumor but also can damage healthy tissue around the	4

Term	Definition	Ref
radiation therapy	tumor. Also known as external beam radiation therapy.	
Physician assistant	Trained professional who has completed an accredited program and is board-certified to perform certain duties of a physician, under the supervision of a licensed physician; some duties include history-taking, physical examination, and minor surgical procedures.	4
Phytochemistry	The biochemical study of plants; concerned with the identification, biosynthesis, metabolism of chemical constituents of plants; especially in regard to natural products.	1
Placebo	A substance that has no active ingredient.	4
Port	A device that is surgically installed to create an opening into the body.	4
Portal vein (hepatic portal vein)	Carries blood to the liver from the spleen, stomach, pancreas, and intestines.	4
Positron emission tomography (PET scan)	Imaging test in which a small amount of radioactive glucose is injected into a vein, a camera detects the radioactivity, and a computer generates detailed images; because cancer cells absorb much more glucose than normal cells, images created by a PET scan can be used to find cancer cells in the pancreas and other parts of the body.	4
Power of attorney	Legal document that appoints a person to make financial decisions for the patient when the patient cannot.	4
Practical Care	A type of hospice care provided by housekeepers, social workers, and volunteers. Practical care covers everything from insurance and other financial matters	2

Term	Definition	Ref
	to routine chores.	
Primary Cancer	A cancer in the organ where it started in. A primary cancer of the pancreas is one that started in the pancreas as opposed to a cancer that started somewhere else and only later spread to the pancreas.	1
Primary Caregiver	See Caregiver.	2
Primary Tumor	The original tumor. In pancreatic cancer, the primary tumor is in the pancreas.	2
Prognosis	The expected pattern and outcome of a disease based on tests.	4
Progression	The growth or spread of cancer after being tested or treated.	4
Protease	An enzyme secreted by the pancreas that breaks down proteins.	2
Protein	A molecule made up of amino acids needed for the body to function properly; proteins are the basis of body structures such as the skin and hair, and of substances such as enzymes.	4
Protocol	A detailed plan of a medical study, treatment, or procedure.	4
Proton beam radiation therapy	Treatment with radiation that uses a stream of positively charged particles that can be focused to reach only the targeted area.	4
Proven therapy	A conventional, traditional, or standard treatment that has been tested and is approved by the Food and Drug Administration.	4
Psychologist	A specialist who can talk with patients and their families about emotional and personal	3

Term	Definition	Ref
	matters and can help them make decisions.	
Pulmonary	Concerning, affecting or associated with the lungs.	3
Pylorus	A thick ring of muscle (a sphincter) between the stomach and duodenum. This sphincter helps control the release of the stomach contents into the small intestine.	4
Pylorus Preserving Pancreatoduodectomy	This is a Modified Whipple Procedure. It involves removal of all or part of the pancreas and the duodenum with preservation of the pylorus (the part of the stomach that connects to the duodenum); usually limited to the head and neck of the pancreas and most often performed for pancreatic carcinoma.	3
Pylorus-preserving Whipple procedure	Surgical procedure in patients with pancreatic cancer that removes most of the duodenum, the head of the pancreas, part of the bile duct, the gallbladder, and lymph nodes in the area of the pancreas; in this procedure, the stomach is spared.	4
Quality of life	The standard of one's well-being.	4
Questionable therapy	Unproven or untested treatments.	4
R0 resection	After surgery to remove a tumor, no tumor remains in the edges of the location where the tumor was removed, either visible to the eye or under a microscope.	4
R1 resection	After surgery to remove a tumor, all the visible tumor was removed but under the microscope there are still visible tumor cells on the edges of the location where the tumor was removed.	4

Term	Definition	Ref
Radiation	The use of energy waves to diagnose or treat disease.	4
Radiation field	The area of the body that receives radiation.	4
Radiation oncologist	A physician trained in treating cancer with high-dose X-rays.	4
Radiation therapy	Also called radiotherapy; treatment of cancer with irradiation.	4
Radioactive	Giving off radiation.	4
Radioactive glucose	Sugar injected into the body to make specific tissue more visible during a PET scan.	4
Radiologist	A physician trained to interpret many different imaging techniques.	4
Radiotherapy	Also called radiation therapy; treatment of cancer with irradiation.	4
Randomization	A method used to prevent bias in research; a computer or a table of random numbers generates treatment assignments, and participants have an equal chance to be assigned to one of two or more groups (e.g., the control group or the investigational group)	3
Randomize	The random or chance assignment of clinical trial participants into different treatment groups; neither the researchers nor the participants can choose which group individuals are placed in. Randomization ensures that groups that will be statistically similar so that the treatments delivered can be compared objectively and without bias.	2
Randomized trial	A clinical trial in which patients are assigned by chance to the different treatments being	4

Term	Definition	Ref
	tested in that trial.	
Recurrence	The reappearance of the cancer after a period of time when it was undetectable. Recurrence can appear in the same place as the primary tumor or in another part of the body.	2
Red blood cell	Oxygen-transporting blood cell.	3
Referring Order	A referral made by the survivor's physician certifying that life expectancy is six months or less if the pancreatic cancer runs its likely course.	2
Regimen	A plan or a regulated course, such as a diet, exercise, or disease treatment, designed to give a good result.	4
Regional anesthesia	A type of drug used for short-term loss of feeling or awareness in a part of the body while awake.	4
Registered Dietitian	A health professional with special training in the use of diet and nutrition to keep the body healthy. A registered dietitian may help the medical team improve the nutritional health of a patient.	3
Relapse	The return of signs and symptoms of a disease after a remission.	4
Remission	The signs and symptoms of cancer have disappeared as a result of treatment.	4
Renal	Relating to or affecting the kidneys.	3
Resect	To surgically remove.	3
Resectable	Cancer that can be surgically removed. In pancreatic cancer, these tumors may lie within the pancreas or extend beyond it, but	4

Term	Definition	Ref
	there is no involvement of the critical arteries or veins in the area. There is no evidence of any spread to areas outside of the tissue removed during a typical surgery for pancreatic cancer.	
Resectable pancreatic cancer	Resectable means that the tumor is able to be removed, or resected, by surgery. This is often the case when the cancer is caught in the early stages and has not grown far outside the pancreas and does not involve other critical structures such as veins and arteries.	3
Resection	Surgery to remove a tumor.	4
Respite Care	A part of hospice care that provides the primary caregiver a short break from caregiving duties while the cancer survivor stays in a hospital facility.	2
Risk factor	Something that increases the chance of developing a disease. Some examples of risk factors for cancer are age, a family history of certain cancers, use of tobacco products, being exposed to radiation or certain chemicals, infection with certain viruses or bacteria, and certain genetic changes.	3
Risk factors	Characteristics, habits, or environmental exposures shown to increase the odds of developing a disease.	4
RNA (ribonucleic acid)	A molecule that carries information for DNA and carries the same genetic code as DNA.	4
Sarcoma	A malignant tumor that looks like connective tissues (bone, cartilage, muscle) under the microscope. Sarcomas are extremely rare in the pancreas.	1

Term	Definition	Ref
Scientific Validity	An objective scientific index by which the accuracy of a test or procedure is measured.	2
SDR	Second Degree Relatives - Aunts, uncles, grandparents, nieces, and nephews	1
Secondary Tumor	A cancerous tumor that has spread from its original site of formation (the primary tumor) to another location in the body. Secondary tumors are treated with the same medical therapies as the primary tumor.	2
Second-line treatment	The next treatment used against a disease when the first treatment fails.	4
Sedative	A drug that helps a person to relax or go to sleep.	4
Seizure	A sudden movement of muscles that cannot be controlled.	2
Sepsis	An infection of the blood. This can be life-threatening and is often treated with antibiotics.	1
Shave biopsy	Surgery to remove a thin tissue sample from the top of a tumor to test for cancer cells.	4
Side effect	A problem that occurs when treatment affects healthy tissues or organs. Some common side effects of cancer treatment are fatigue, pain, nausea, vomiting, decreased blood cell counts, hair loss, and mouth sores.	3
Signs	Any objective evidence of a disease, for example, evidence perceptible to the examining physician. (See also Symptoms.)	4
Single-agent drug	A drug that is used as the only treatment.	4
Small intestine	The part of the digestive tract that is located	3

Term	Definition	Ref
	between the stomach and the large intestine.	
Social Worker	A professional trained to talk with people and their families about emotional or physical needs, and to find them support services.	3
Soluble Fiber	A digestible fiber that dissolves readily in water. Food sources include fruits, vegetables, legumes, seeds, oats, barley, and rye. Additionally, over-the-counter products that contain soluble fiber are available. Possible health effects include lowered blood cholesterol, slowed glucose absorption, slowing transit time of food through the upper gastrointestinal tract, and bulking of stool.	2
Somatuline Depot (lanreotide acetate)	One of the approved drugs for treating symptoms of pancreatic neuroendocrine tumors.	4
Sonogram	A computer picture of areas inside the body, created by sound waves bounced off tissues and organs.	4
Spleen	An organ located on the left side of the abdomen, near the stomach, which is part of the lymphatic system; it produces white blood cells, filters the blood, stores blood cells, and destroys old blood cells.	4
Splenic artery	The blood vessel that brings oxygenated blood to the spleen. It branches from the celiac artery.	4
Splenic vein	Drains blood from the spleen, part of the stomach, and part of the pancreas.	4
Squamous Cell	A cell that flattens out as it grows. This type of cell usually lines the inside of ducts in	2

Term	Definition	Ref
	human organs.	
Stage	In cancer, the stage denotes the extent of the disease, especially whether it has spread from the original site to other parts of the body.	4
Staging	Staging describes the extent or severity of a person's cancer based on the size of the primary tumor, lymph node involvement, and if the tumor has spread to other organs. Stages range from the tumor being localized without anything spreading in stage I to a tumor that has spread outside its primary origin, or stage IV. Knowing the stage of disease helps the doctor plan treatment.	3
Staging cancer	A standardized way to classify a tumor based on its size, whether it has spread, and where it has spread; staging measures the extent of the disease.	4
Standard of care	The process that a healthcare professional should follow to treat a medical problem.	4
Standard Treatment	The treatment that is widely used in the medical community for a given stage of disease. The standard treatment may also be the standard of care.	2
Steatorrhea	Excessive amounts of fat in the stool. Sometimes this can appear as an oil slick on top of the toilet water after the patient has had a bowel movement.	4
Stem cell	Parent cell that grows and divides to produce red blood cells, white blood cells, and platelets. Found primarily in the bone marrow, but also in the peripheral blood.	3
Stem cell	Therapeutic procedure in which bone marrow or peripheral blood stem cells are	3

Term	Definition	Ref
transplantation	collected, stored, and infused into a patient following high-dose chemotherapy to restore blood cell production.	
Stent	Device placed in a body structure (such as the pancreatic duct) to keep it open.	4
Stereotactic body radiation therapy (SBRT)	Multiple beams of high-dose radiation focused on a specified location in the body. The technique enables the radiation oncologist to kill cancer cells and limit the exposure of healthy tissue to radiation.	4
Stroma	A kind of framework, made up of connective tissue, which provides support, structure, and anchoring for organs.	4
Subcutaneous	Under the skin.	4
Sunitinib (Sutent®)	A targeted therapy drug approved in 2011 by the FDA to treat advanced pancreatic neuroendocrine tumors. It may help slow or prevent cancer cells from multiplying and dividing. It may also slow the formation of blood vessels that provide nutrients and oxygen to the tumor.	2
Sunitinib malate (Sutent)	One of the approved chemotherapy drugs for pancreatic neuroendocrine tumors, it is a tyrosine kinase inhibitor with potential anticancer activity.	4
Superior mesenteric artery	A major blood vessel for the intestines, colon, duodenum, and part of the pancreas. It branches off of the abdominal aorta.	4
Superior mesenteric vein	The blood vessel that drains the small intestine. Its endpoint is behind the head of the pancreas.	4
Supplement	A product that is added to the diet, such as a	4

Term	Definition	Ref
	vitamin, mineral, or herb.	
Supportive care	In patients with cancer, use of medications to prevent or counteract unwanted side effects of cancer or its treatment to increase quality of life.	4
Surgeon	A doctor who removes or repairs a part of the body by operating on the patient.	3
Surgery	A procedure to remove or repair a part of the body or to find out whether disease is present. An operation.	3
Surgical oncologist	A doctor who is an expert in cancer surgery.	4
Surgical staging	Procedures done during surgery that are used to find out how far cancer has spread.	4
Surveillance	Follow-up testing that is done after treatment ends to look for new tumors.	4
Survivor	A term used to describe any person who has been diagnosed with cancer, no matter how long it has been since the diagnosis. Definitions vary throughout the cancer community and are best-defined by the individual.	2
Symptom	An indication that a person has a condition or disease. Some examples of symptoms for pancreatic cancer include jaundice, weight loss, fatigue, nausea, vomiting, and pain.	2
Systemic treatment	In cancer, a treatment in which a drug enters and travels throughout the body to reach tumor cells.	4
Tail of the pancreas	The thin tip of the organ in the left part of the abdomen, near the spleen.	4
Tarceva (erlotinib	One of the approved chemotherapy drugs	4

Term	Definition	Ref
hydrochloride)	for pancreatic cancer, it is a receptor kinase inhibitor and prevents cancer cells from multiplying.	
Targeted therapy	Treatment designed to kill only cancer cells and not healthy cells.	4
TDR	Third Degree Relatives - First cousins, great-aunts, and uncles	1
Therapy	The treatment of disease.	4
Three-dimensional conformal radiation therapy (3D-CRT)	Treatment with radiation that uses beams matched to the shape of the tumor.	4
Thrombophlebitis	An inflammation of the veins accompanied by thrombus formation. It is sometimes referred to as Trousseau's sign.	1
Thrombus	A clot within the blood vessels. It may occlude (block) the vessel or may be attached to the wall of the vessel without blocking the blood flow.	1
Tissue	A group or layer of cells that work together to perform a specific function.	3
TNM system	A system used to evaluate cancer; T stands for tumor, N for node, and M for metastasis.	4
Total pancreatectomy	Procedure now seldom used to remove the entire pancreas and spleen in patients with pancreatic cancer.	4
Toxicity	The degree to which a substance can harm humans or animals.	4
Transdermal	Through the skin.	4
Transducer	A hand-held tool that bounces sound waves off tissue to make pictures of the inside of	4

Term	Definition	Ref
	the body.	
Translational research	Takes findings from basic science to enhance human health and well-being. This is done by applying discoveries generated during research in the laboratory and in preclinical studies to the development of trials and studies in humans.	3
Treatment plan	A written course of action through cancer treatment and beyond.	4
Tumor	An abnormal mass of tissue. Tumors are a classic sign of inflammation and can be benign or malignant (cancerous).	4
Tumor extension	How far the tumor has grown into nearby tissue.	4
Tumor grade	How closely the cancer cells look like normal cells.	4
Tumor Marker	A substance found in tissue, blood, or other body fluids that may be a sign of cancer or certain benign (noncancerous) conditions. Most tumor markers are made by both normal cells and cancer cells, but they are made in larger amounts by cancer cells.	3
Tumor regression	A decrease in the size of the tumor.	4
U.S. Food and Drug Administration (FDA)	A federal government agency that regulates drugs and food in the United States.	4
Ultrasonography	Also called a sonogram, ultrasonogram, or ultrasound scan; imaging method that bounces sound waves off internal organs to produce echoes; a computer creates patterns from these echoes that can determine whether tissue is normal or abnormal.	4

Term	Definition	Ref
Ultrasound	A procedure in which high-energy sound waves are bounced off internal tissues or organs and make echoes. The echo patterns are shown on the screen of an ultrasound machine, forming a picture of body tissues called a sonogram. Also called ultrasonography.	3
Uncinate process of the pancreas	The part of the gland that bends backwards and underneath the body of the pancreas. Two very important blood vessels, the superior mesenteric artery and vein, cross in front of this part of the pancreas.	4
Unconventional therapy	Term used to cover all types of complementary and alternative treatments that fall outside of proven therapies. (See also Alternative therapy.)	4
Unresectable	Cancer that has grown beyond the pancreas and has invaded vital structures around the pancreas. Unresectable cancer cannot be entirely removed by surgery.	4
Upper gastrointestinal (GI) endoscopy	A process in which a thin, long tool is guided into the esophagus and stomach.	4
Vaccine	A biological agent inserted into the body to prevent a disease.	4
Vaccine therapy	A treatment used to help the body's disease-fighting ability (immune system) prevent a disease.	4
Vital organ	A functional group of tissue in the body that is needed to live.	4
Vitamin	A nutrient essential in small amounts to help the body's metabolic reactions occur properly.	2

Term	Definition	Ref
Whipple procedure	Surgical procedure in patients with pancreatic cancer that removes part of the stomach, the duodenum, the head of the pancreas, part of the bile duct, the gallbladder, and lymph nodes in the area of the pancreas.	4
White blood cell	Also called a leukocyte. One of the major cell types in the blood. Responsible for immune defenses.	3
Widespread metastatic disease	Cancer that has spread from the first tumor to many distant locations in the body.	4
Will	Legal document that describes how a person wants his or her money and property divided after death.	4
Xeloda (capecitabine)	One of the approved chemotherapy drugs for pancreatic cancer, it gets metabolized into 5-FU; in either form the drug disrupts the cell replication cycle.	4
X-ray	High-energy radiation with waves shorter than those of visible light, used in low doses to make images that help to diagnose diseases and in high doses to treat cancer.	4

About the Author

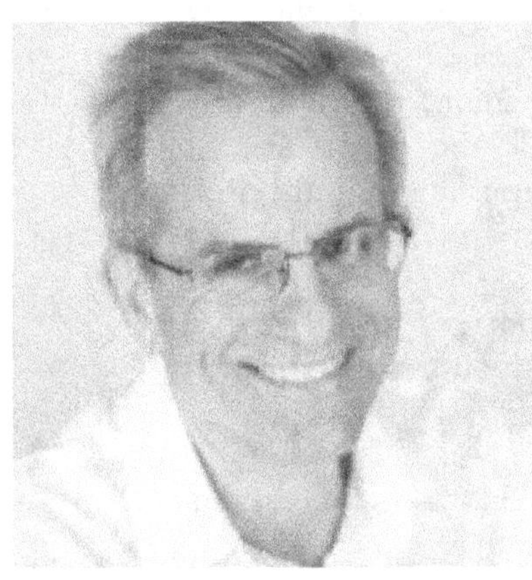

Robert Koshinskie is the author of two books on Modern Devil's Advocacy, "Devils in the Details" and "Modern Devil's Advocacy" (https://amzn.to/3JtxwsB).

He was a mentor in the NSF Innovation Corps (I-Corps™) Program working with a University of North Carolina (UNCG), Greensboro I-Corps™ team for the development of a novel medical device.[193]

He created and ran a critical thinking and decision-making seminar through the North Carolina State University (NCSU), Raleigh Division of Continuing and Professional Education.

If you have questions, comments, or find errors in this book that need to be fixed, then please don't hesitate to reach out to me on LinkedIn https://www.linkedin.com/in/robertkoshinskie/

- LinkedIn Messaging – Overview, https://bit.ly/3yyQjjI
- How to Send an InMail Message, https://bit.ly/3OXt1t7

ENDNOTES

I state the original date for published references below when available, otherwise, the reference date stated is the date when I accessed the material on the web.

---

[1] Whipple Procedure, John Hopkins Medicine, 13 August 2022, https://www.hopkinsmedicine.org/health/conditions-and-diseases/pancreatic-cancer/whipple-procedure

[2] Steven Merlin, Hematology/Oncology Pharmacy Association, 27 July 2022, https://www.hoparx.org/patient-outreach/steve-merlin

[3] LGBT glossary: An A-Z Of LGBTQ+ Terms, Casey Tanner, Flo Health, 17 December 2021, https://flo.health/lgbtq/lgbt-glossary

[4] What is Cancer, The National Cancer Institute, 18 June 2022, https://www.cancer.gov/about-cancer/understanding/what-is-cancer

[5] What causes cancer?, Stanford Healthcare, 20 June 2022, https://stanfordhealthcare.org/medical-conditions/cancer/cancer/cancer-causes.html

[6] One Organ, Two Different Functions, Johns Hopkins, 25 June 2022, https://pathology.jhu.edu/pancreas/basics/function

[7] The Anatomy of the Duodenum, Verywell Health, Sherry Christiansen, 22 February 2022, https://www.verywellhealth.com/duodenum-anatomy-4780308

[8] What is the function of bile?, MedicineNet, 2 February 2021, https://www.medicinenet.com/what_is_the_function_of_bile/article.htm

[9] Liver: Anatomy and Functions, John Hopkins, 25 June 2022, https://www.hopkinsmedicine.org/health/conditions-and-diseases/liver-anatomy-and-functions

[10] Controlling Weight Loss, The Pancreatic Cancer Action Network, 18 June 2022, https://www.pancan.org/facing-pancreatic-cancer/living-with-pancreatic-cancer/diet-and-nutrition/controlling-weight-loss/

[11] Cancer Stat Facts: Pancreatic Cancer, Cancer Stat Facts: Pancreatic Cancer, 16 July 2022, https://seer.cancer.gov/statfacts/html/pancreas.html

[12] Pancreatic Cancer Facts, Hirshberg Foundation for Pancreatic Cancer Research, 29 July 2022, https://pancreatic.org/pancreatic-cancer/pancreatic-cancer-facts/

[13] Survival Rates for Pancreatic Cancer, American Cancer Society, 23 July 2022, https://www.cancer.org/cancer/pancreatic-cancer/detection-diagnosis-staging/survival-rates.html

[14] Whipple Procedure, the Mayo Clinic, 9 August 2022, https://www.mayoclinic.org/tests-procedures/whipple-procedure/about/pac-20385054

[15] Pancreatic cancer specialist explains challenges of the disease and treatment advances, The Conversation, 31 May 2019, https://bit.ly/3bRXbjm

[16] Long-Term Trends in SEER Age-Adjusted Incidence Rates, 1975-2019 Observed SEER Incidence Rate by Cancer Site, Both Sexes, All Races, All Ages, NIH, 13 July 2022, https://bit.ly/3yy0xzw

[17] SEER 5-Year Relative Survival Rates, 2012-2018, All Stages by Cancer Site, Both Sexes, All Races, All Ages, NIH, 13 July 2022, https://bit.ly/3IyqlQN

[18] Gaddam S, Abboud Y, Oh J, Samaan JS, Nissen NN, Lu SC, Lo SK. Incidence of Pancreatic Cancer by Age and Sex in the US, 2000-2018. JAMA. 2021 Nov 23;326(20):2075-2077. doi: 10.1001/jama.2021.18859. PMID: 34689206; PMCID: PMC8543346.

[19] What's New in Pancreatic Cancer Treatment, Kim Reiss Binder, MD, YouTube, 5 October 2021, https://youtu.be/l1HCPjUBm1s

[20] Gemcitabine, MedlinePlus, 23 July 2022, https://www.cancer.gov/about-cancer/treatment/drugs/gemcitabinehydrochloride

[21] Folfirinox, MedlinePlus, 23 July 2022, https://www.cancer.gov/about-cancer/treatment/drugs/folfirinox

[22] CA 19-9 Blood Test (Pancreatic Cancer), Mayo Clinic, 20 June 2022, https://medlineplus.gov/lab-tests/ca-19-9-blood-test-pancreatic-cancer/

[23] Abdominal ultrasound for pancreatic cancer, Cancer Research UK, 20 June 2022, https://www.cancerresearchuk.org/about-cancer/pancreatic-cancer/getting-diagnosed/tests/abdominal-ultrasound

[24] CT Scan, Mayo Clinic, 19 June 2022, https://www.mayoclinic.org/tests-procedures/ct-scan/about/pac-20393675

[25] MRI Scan, Mayo Clinic, 19 June 2022, https://www.mayoclinic.org/tests-procedures/mri/about/pac-20384768

[26] Endoscope, Merriam-Webster, 20 June 2022, https://www.merriam-webster.com/dictionary/endoscope

[27] Upper endoscopy, Mayo Clinic, 20 June 2022, https://www.mayoclinic.org/tests-procedures/endoscopy/about/pac-20395197

[28] Endoscopic ultrasound, Mayo Clinic, 25 June 2002, https://mayocl.in/3y3vJ9q

[29] Endoscopic Retrograde Cholangiopancreatography (ERCP), National Institute of Diabetes and Digestive and Kidney Diseases (NIDDK), 25 June 2022, https://www.niddk.nih.gov/health-information/diagnostic-tests/endoscopic-retrograde-cholangiopancreatography#perform

[30] What Is an Infusion Pump?, Food and Drug Administration, 13 December 2017, https://www.fda.gov/medical-devices/infusion-pumps/what-infusion-pump

[31] *Collaterals* are new vessels that the body creates in order to bypass an obstruction to blood flow.

[32] What are some of the limitations and potential harms of the PSA test for prostate cancer screening?, National Cancer Institute, 2 July 2022, https://bit.ly/3OSwedk

[33] Ruth Bader Ginsburg's Pancreatic Cancer Found Early, WebMD Cancer Center, 13 February 2009, https://www.webmd.com/cancer/pancreatic-cancer/news/20090213/ruth-bader-ginsburgs-pancreatic-cancer-found-early

[34] What You Need to Know About Pancreatic Enzymes, Deborah Gerszberg, Columbia Surgery, 30 June 2022, https://columbiasurgery.org/news/2013/12/20/what-you-need-know-about-pancreatic-enzymes

[35] Side effects of chemotherapy, Canadian Cancer Society, 25 June 2002, https://bit.ly/3OCrSHv

[36] Chemo brain, Mayo Clinic, 26 June 2022, https://www.mayoclinic.org/diseases-conditions/chemo-brain/symptoms-causes/syc-20351060

37 How Effective Is Magic Mouthwash?, Healthline, 7 January 2022,
https://www.healthline.com/health/magic-mouthwash#takeaway
38 Oral thrush, Mayo Clinic, 27 July 2022, https://www.mayoclinic.org/diseases-conditions/oral-thrush/symptoms-causes/syc-20353533
39 Nystatin, MedlinePlus, 15 December 2018,
https://medlineplus.gov/druginfo/meds/a682758.html
40 CeraVe moisturizing cream,
https://www.cerave.com/skincare/moisturizers/moisturizing-cream
41 Raynaud's Phenomenon, John's Hopkins Medicine, 4 July 2022,
https://www.hopkinsmedicine.org/health/conditions-and-diseases/raynauds-phenomenon
42 Raynaud's disease, Mayo Clinic, 26 June 2022, https://www.mayoclinic.org/diseases-conditions/raynauds-disease/symptoms-causes/syc-20363571
43 It's Time to Revisit the High Knees Exercise You Learned in PE, Healthline, 15 July 2022, https://www.healthline.com/health/fitness/high-knees-benefits#muscles-worked
44 How to Do Chair Squats Like a Pro, Even If You're a Beginner, 15 July 2022,
https://greatist.com/fitness/chair-squats
45 How using a resistance band can take your bicep curl to the next level, Stephanie Mansour, Today, 4 November 2022, https://www.today.com/health/these-resistance-band-exercises-will-make-your-bicep-curls-more-t237582
46 Standing Decline Chest Press Using Resistance Bands, Home Gym Fitness Channel, YouTube, 21 December 2018, https://www.youtube.com/watch?v=4iVpEZ-Vl8U
47 Letter writing kit examples https://amzn.to/3ukuUIz , https://amzn.to/3a8yWwP , https://amzn.to/3OBprVI
48 Field listings -Religion, CIA Factbook, 27 June 2022, https://www.cia.gov/the-world-factbook/field/religions/
49 Religion, Pew Research Center, 4 July 2022,
https://www.pewresearch.org/topic/religion/
50 Religion, Dictionary.com, 25 June 2022,
https://www.dictionary.com/browse/religion
51 The Baltimore Catechism, Revised Edition (1941),
https://www.catholicity.com/baltimore-catechism/
52 Why Do We Cover Crucifixes and Statues During Lent?, Philip Kosloski, Catholic Education Resource Center (CERC), 29 June 2022, https://bit.ly/3yAd7zr
53 Monstrance, Merriam-Webster, 16 July 2022, https://www.merriam-webster.com/dictionary/monstrance
54 Monstrance, The Word is Catholic, 29 June 2022,
https://www.thewordiscatholic.com/the-monstrance
55 Atheist, Merriam-Webster, 18 June 2022, https://www.merriam-webster.com/dictionary/atheist
56 What is an Agnostic by Bertrand Russell, Scepsis Magazine, 18 June 2022,
https://scepsis.net/eng/articles/id_5.php
57 The Jefferson Bible, 13 August 2022, http://thejeffersonbible.com/
58 The Founding Fathers, Deism, and Christianity, David L. Holmes, Encyclopaedia Britannica, 13 August 2022, https://www.britannica.com/topic/The-Founding-

Fathers-Deism-and-Christianity-1272214

59 The Faith of the Founding Fathers, Dr. Gregg Frazer, The Master's University, 4 October 2016, https://www.masters.edu/news/the-faith-of-the-founding-fathers.html

60 John 19:15, BibleGateway, 27 June 2022, https://www.biblegateway.com/passage/?search=John+19%3A15&version=ESV

61 Biblical Contradictions, American Atheists, 27 June 2022, https://www.atheists.org/activism/resources/biblical-contradictions/

62 Bart Ehrman's author page, Amazon.com, 27 June 2022, https://amzn.to/3y9eXWA

63 Who chose the books of the Bible?, Alice Camille, US Catholic, 21 March 2012, https://uscatholic.org/articles/201203/who-decided-which-books-made-it-into-the-bible/

64 The Gospels, Rebecca Denova, World History Encyclopedia, 26 February 2021, https://www.worldhistory.org/The_Gospels/

65 Apologetics, Catholic Answers, Charles F. Aiken, 18 June 2022, https://www.catholic.com/encyclopedia/apologetics

66 The Task of the Christian Apologist, Article: DT253, Christian Research Institute (CRI), Charlotte, NC, 27 June 2022, https://www.equip.org/PDF/DT253.pdf

67 Hypothesis, Merriam-Webster Dictionary, 2 July 2022, https://www.merriam-webster.com/dictionary/hypothesis

68 Null Hypothesis, CFI Education Inc., 7 May 2022, https://corporatefinanceinstitute.com/resources/knowledge/other/null-hypothesis-2/

69 Theory, Merriam-Webster Dictionary, 2 July 2022, https://www.merriam-webster.com/dictionary/theory

70 Transcript of Ken Ham vs Bill Nye Debate, Written by Bill Browning, 10 February 2014, https://www.youngearth.org/index.php/archives/rmcf-articles/item/21-transcript-of-ken-ham-vs-bill-nye-debate

71 Bill Nye Debates Ken Ham - HD (Official), YouTube, 27 June 2022, https://youtu.be/z6kgvhG3AkI

72 Was Giordano Bruno Burned at the Stake for Believing in Exoplanets?, Alberto A. Martínez, Scientific American, 19 March 2018, https://blogs.scientificamerican.com/observations/was-giordano-bruno-burned-at-the-stake-for-believing-in-exoplanets/

73 Christopher Clavius, Society of Catholic Scientists, 28 June 2022, https://catholicscientists.org/scientists-of-the-past/christopher-clavius/

74 Christopher Clavius, The Galileo Project, 28 June 2022, http://galileo.rice.edu/sci/clavius.html

75 The Jesuit astronomer who conceived of the Big Bang, Korey Haynes, Scientific American, 12 October 2018, https://astronomy.com/news/2018/10/the-jesuit-astronomer-who-conceived-of-the-big-bang

76 Francis Collins, M.D., Ph.D., NIH National Human Genome Research Institute, 27 June 2022, https://www.genome.gov/staff/Francis-S-Collins-MD-PhD

77 Dark Energy, Dark Matter, NASA Science, https://science.nasa.gov/astrophysics/focus-areas/what-is-dark-energy

78 Bronze Age, History, 29 June 2022, https://www.history.com/topics/pre-history/bronze-age

79 Iron Age, History, 29 June 2022, https://www.history.com/topics/pre-history/iron-

age

[80] The Varieties of Scientific Experience, Carl Sagan, Penguin Books, ISBN-13: 978-0143112624, 6 November 2007, https://amzn.to/3yyR7Fg

[81] Carl Sagan interview with Charlie Rose, 27 May 1996, https://youtu.be/U8HEwO-2L4w

[82] Richard Feynman and the Pleasure Principle, Algis Valiunas, The New Atlantis, Spring 2018, https://www.thenewatlantis.com/publications/richard-feynman-and-the-pleasure-principle

[83] What Is Intelligent Design?, Intelligent Design, 27 June 2022, https://intelligentdesign.org/whatisid/

[84] A Scientific History – and Philosophical Defense – of the Theory of Intelligent Design, Stephen C. Meyer, Ph.D., https://intelligentdesign.org/articles/a-scientific-history-and-philosophical-defense-of-the-theory-of-intelligent-design/

[85] 'I crossed over': Survivors of near-death experiences share 'afterlife' stories, Lindsay Sobel Dyner, Chris Serico, TODAY, 15 July2016, https://www.today.com/health/i-crossed-over-survivors-near-death-experiences-share-afterlife-stories-t12841

[86] 'Afterlives': 40 Stories Of What Follows Death, NPR Talk of the Nation, 17 February 17, https://www.npr.org/templates/story/story.php?storyId=100778241

[87] I died and came back to life, 'heaven' was incredible I can't wait to go back, Lauren Windle, The U.S. Sun, 8 August 2022, https://www.the-sun.com/lifestyle/5954436/died-came-back-life-heaven-incredible/

[88] The Ongoing Mystery of Jesus's Face, https://www.history.com/news/what-did-jesus-look-like

[89] Confirmation bias, Britannica, 18 August 2022, https://www.britannica.com/science/confirmation-bias

[90] Key Thinkers: Michael Persinger, Philosophy Dungeon, 2 July 2022, https://philosophydungeon.weebly.com/scholar-persinger.html

[91] God Helmet Experiment, Elixir of Knowledge, 1 July 2015, https://www.elixirofknowledge.com/2015/07/god-helmet-experiment.html

[92] This Is Your Brain on God, Jack Hitt, Wired, 1 November 1999, https://www.wired.com/1999/11/persinger/

[93] The 'God Helmet' and neuro-spirituality, Assoc. Prof. Dr. Syed Alwi Shahab, International Conference on Modern Approach in Humanities, Kuala Lumpur, Malaysia, 14 December 2015, https://bit.ly/3y4EJLu

[94] God on the Brain; The God Helmet and How We Experience the Divine, Lisa Trank, August 23, 2019, https://www.gaia.com/article/god-on-the-brain-the-god-helmet-and-how-we-experience-the-divine

[95] Magnet therapy brings hope to people with depression, Today, 6 July 2022 https://www.today.com/video/how-magnet-therapy-can-help-treat-depression-143573573760

[96] SAINT: Hope for new treatment of depression, Deirdre Cohen, Ed Givnish, CBS News, 7 November 2021, https://www.cbsnews.com/news/saint-treatment-for-depression/

[97] Prayer and healing: A medical and scientific perspective on randomized controlled trials, Chittaranjan Andrade, Rajiv Radhakrishnan, Indian J Psychiatry. 2009 Oct-Dec; 51(4): 247–253, doi: 10.4103/0019-5545.58288

98 Have Christians Accepted the Scientific Conclusion That God Does Not Answer Intercessory Prayer?, Brian Bolton, Free Inquiry, Volume 39, No. 1, Dec18/Jan19, https://secularhumanism.org/2018/12/have-christians-accepted-the-scientific-conclusion-that-god-does-not-answer-intercessory-prayer/

99 Largest Study of Prayer to Date Finds It Has No Power to Heal, Denise Gellene, Thomas H. Maugh II, Los Angeles Times, 31 March 2006, https://www.latimes.com/archives/la-xpm-2006-mar-31-sci-prayer31-story.html

100 What Is Intercessory Prayer? - Example and Meaning, Candice Lucey, Christianity.com, 16 July 2020, https://www.christianity.com/wiki/prayer/what-is-intercessory-prayer.html

101 Miracles, Prayer, Faith – A Marian Shrine's Perfect Trio, Joseph Pronechen, National Catholic Register, 10 July 2022, https://www.ncregister.com/features/miracles-prayer-faith-a-marian-shrine-s-perfect-trio

102 Does Prayer Influence God?, Charles Stanley, Sermons Online, 14 August 2022, https://youtu.be/MsSuhpXxttY

103 Mireille Mathieu - Ave Maria (Official Video), YouTube, 1November 2018, https://youtu.be/ZUUXbc9aVv4

104 Gregorian Chant: Kyrie Eleison, YouTube, 14 March 2012, https://youtu.be/FV-L5sg6yMI

105 Hark the herald angels sing, The Choir of King's College, Cambridge, YouTube, 28 July 2008, https://youtu.be/shr4O1qGXB4

106 Gregory Porter - Take Me To The Alley, YouTube, 6 May 2016, https://youtu.be/Qj5z4SbrH20

107 Prosperity Theology, David Jeremiah, Christianity Today, 4 July 2022, https://www.christianitytoday.com/biblestudies/articles/theology/prosperitytheology.html

108 Mockingbird (quotes), IMDB, 11 July, 2022, https://www.imdb.com/title/tt3060876/

109 What is Philosophy?, The Philosophy Foundation, 27 June 2022, https://www.philosophy-foundation.org/what-is-philosophy

110 Ryan Holiday, Amazon Author Page, 27 June 2022, https://amzn.to/3nxIJiV

111 Epictetus, Stanford Encyclopedia of Philosophy, 15 June 2021, https://plato.stanford.edu/entries/epictetus/

112 Marcus Aurelius, Stanford Encyclopedia of Philosophy, 22 December 2017, https://plato.stanford.edu/entries/marcus-aurelius/

113 Seneca, Stanford Encyclopedia of Philosophy, 15 January 2020, https://plato.stanford.edu/entries/seneca/

114 Stoic Philosophy as a Cognitive-Behavioral Therapy, Donald Robertson, 12 February 2019, https://donaldrobertson.name/2019/02/12/stoic-philosophy-as-a-cognitive-behavioral-therapy/

115 The Philosophical Foundations of Cognitive Behavioral Therapy, Edward Murgia, Kim Diaz, Journal of Evidence-Based Psychotherapies, Vol. 15, No. 1, March 2015, 37-50, https://philpapers.org/archive/DIATPF.pdf

116 Stoic, Merriam-Webster, 27, June 2022, https://www.merriam-webster.com/dictionary/stoic

117 What is the origin of stoic?, Merriam-Webster, 27, June 2022, https://www.merriam-

webster.com/dictionary/stoic#note-1
[118] Taoism, National Geographic, 20 May 2022,
https://education.nationalgeographic.org/resource/taoism
[119] Tao, Merriam-Webster, 18 June 2022, https://www.merriam-webster.com/dictionary/Tao
[120] Lao-Tzu, Joshua J. Mark, World History Encyclopedia, 9 July 2020,
https://www.worldhistory.org/Lao-Tzu/
[121] Tao Te Ching, Lao-tzu (Translation by Stephen. Mitchell), 20 July 1995,
http://albanycomplementaryhealth.com/wp-content/uploads/2016/07/TaoTeChing-LaoTzu-StephenMitchellTranslation-33p.pdf
[122] TANG SOO DO, American Tang Soo Do Association, 27 July 2022,
https://americantangsoodoassociation.net/tang-soo-do/
[123] The History of Aikido, Aikido Association of America & Aikido Association
International, 27 July 2022, https://aaa-aikido.com/history-of-aikido/
[124] The History of Aikido, The MIT Aikido Club, 27 July 2022,
https://aikido.mit.edu/history-aikido
[125] Theories of Ageing, Physiopedia, 24 June 2022, https://bit.ly/3adg4wE
[126] Senescence, NIH National Cancer Institute, 29 June 2022,
https://www.cancer.gov/publications/dictionaries/cancer-terms/def/senescence
[127] Compression of Morbidity Theory, Stanford School of Medicine, 24 June 2022,
https://palliative.stanford.edu/overview-of-palliative-care/compression-of-morbidity-theory/
[128] Will CPR Save Your Life? Probably Not, Study Says, Steven Reinberg, WebMD
HealthDay News, 17 July 17 2020, https://www.webmd.com/first-aid/news/20200717/will-cpr-save-your-life-probably-not-study-says
[129] Wild Mouse POV at Hershey Park video, 13 January 2014,
https://youtu.be/JNzDq-dlzts
[130] Good Will Hunting, IMSDB Movie Scripts, 24 June 2022,
https://imsdb.com/scripts/Good-Will-Hunting.html
[131] Jackie, IMDB, 20 June 2022, https://www.imdb.com/title/tt1619029/
[132] Jesuit apologizes to Camelot, The Georgetown Voice, 4 December 2003,
https://georgetownvoice.com/2003/12/04/jesuit-apologizes-to-camelot/
[133] The Kennedys' Jesuit, The Georgetown Voice, 15 January 2004,
https://georgetownvoice.com/2004/01/15/the-kennedys-jesuit/
[134] Zoe Clark Coates MBE's Personal Story, Saying Goodbye, 29 July 2022,
https://www.sayinggoodbye.org/about/people/zoes-story/
[135] LinkedIn post by Rachel Mae, 23 June 2022,
https://www.linkedin.com/feed/update/urn:li:activity:6945737409917591552/
[136] Live Like You're Dying, Outside Magazine, 29 June 2022,
https://www.outsideonline.com/video/live-like-youre-dying-the-story-of-one-skateboarders-battle-with-cancer/
[137] Diane Ronnau, veteran CBS News producer, passes away, CBS News, 23 July 2022,
https://www.cbsnews.com/news/diane-ronnau-veteran-cbs-news-producer-passes-away/
[138] Eye To Eye: Diane Ronnau's Fight Against Cancer (CBS News), 29 March 2007,
https://youtu.be/tgyb4GLsxIg

[139] George Edward Pelham Box, MacTutor, 18 July 2022, https://mathshistory.st-andrews.ac.uk/Biographies/Box/

[140] Robert Duran has stage 4 pancreatic cancer but uses biking as a way to heal, raise awareness, Emily Alvarenga, San Diego Union-Tribune, 16 June 2022, https://bit.ly/3NAEGwN

[141] Eight-year Survivor's Success with Precision Medicine and a Clinical Trial, Jennifer Kennedy, Pancreatic Cancer Action Network, 10 June 2020, https://www.pancan.org/stories/survivors/eight-year-survivors-success-with-precision-medicine-and-a-clinical-trial/

[142] Deadly cancer quickly shrinks by 50% with 'one-and-done' therapy: study, Adriana Diaz, New York Post, 3 June 2022, https://nypost.com/2022/06/03/deadly-cancer-quickly-shrinks-by-50-with-one-and-done-therapy-study/

[143] I'll Never Stop Fighting, Lynne Holcomb, Let's Win! Pancreatic Cancer, 22 August, 2019, https://letswinpc.org/my-treatment/2019/08/22/never-stop-fighting-for-clinical-trial/

[144] Jack London, Bartleby, 16 July 2022, https://www.bartleby.com/73/1118.html

[145] 'Shuffle Off This Mortal Coil' Meaning, No Sweat Shakespeare, 13 July 2022, https://nosweatshakespeare.com/quotes/famous/mortal-coil/

[146] Living wills and advance directives for medical decisions, Mayo Clinic, 22 June 2022, https://www.mayoclinic.org/healthy-lifestyle/consumer-health/in-depth/living-wills/art-20046303

[147] Advance Care Planning: Health Care Directives, National Institute on Aging, 22 June 2022, https://www.nia.nih.gov/health/advance-care-planning-health-care-directives

[148] Advance Health Care Directives and POLST, Family Caregiver Alliance, 22 June 2022, https://www.caregiver.org/resource/advance-health-care-directives-and-polst/

[149] Living Will, Mayo Clinic, 22 June 2022, https://www.mayoclinic.org/healthy-lifestyle/consumer-health/in-depth/living-wills/art-20046303

[150] Advance Health Care Directives and POLST, Family Caregiver Alliance, 22 June 2022, https://www.caregiver.org/resource/advance-health-care-directives-and-polst/

[151] Oxaliplatin Injection, Medline Plus, 20 June 2022, https://medlineplus.gov/druginfo/meds/a607035.html

[152] Irinotecan Injection, MedlinePlus, 20 June 2022, https://medlineplus.gov/druginfo/meds/a608043.html

[153] Fluorouracil (5FU), Cancer Research UK, 20 June 2022, https://www.cancerresearchuk.org/about-cancer/cancer-in-general/treatment/cancer-drugs/drugs/fluorouracil

[154] CAR T Cells: Engineering Patients' Immune Cells to Treat Their Cancers, National Cancer Institute, 23 June 2022, https://www.cancer.gov/about-cancer/treatment/research/car-t-cells

[155] Can mRNA Vaccines Help Treat Cancer?, National Cancer Institute, 20 January 2022, https://www.cancer.gov/news-events/cancer-currents-blog/2022/mrna-vaccines-to-treat-cancer

[156] Scientists find the cause of most common pancreatic cancer, Knowridge Science Report, 13 June 2022, https://knowridge.com/2022/06/scientists-find-the-cause-of-most-common-pancreatic-cancer/

[157] Chemotherapy Safety, The American Cancer Society, 22 June 2022,

https://www.cancer.org/treatment/treatments-and-side-effects/treatment-types/chemotherapy/chemotherapy-safety.html

[158] Cancer-Causing Substances in the Environment, National Cancer Institute, 10 July 2022, https://www.cancer.gov/about-cancer/causes-prevention/risk/substances

[159] 'Disturbing': weedkiller ingredient tied to cancer found in 80% of US urine samples, Carey Gillam, The Guardian, 9 July 2022, https://www.theguardian.com/us-news/2022/jul/09/weedkiller-glyphosate-cdc-study-urine-samples

[160] Drug Disposal: FDA's Flush List for Certain Medicines, US Food and Drug Administration (FDA), 1 October 2020, https://www.fda.gov/drugs/disposal-unused-medicines-what-you-should-know/drug-disposal-fdas-flush-list-certain-medicines

[161] Drugs in the water, Harvard Health Publishing, 1 June 2011, https://www.health.harvard.edu/newsletter_article/drugs-in-the-water

[162] Controlled Substance Public Disposal Locations, Drug Enforcement Administration, 25 June 2022, https://apps.deadiversion.usdoj.gov/pubdispsearch/spring/main?execution=e2s1

[163] Drugs in the water, Harvard Health Publishing, 1 June 2011, https://www.health.harvard.edu/newsletter_article/drugs-in-the-water

[164] The Law of Unintended Consequences, Farnam Street, 7 July 2022, https://fs.blog/unintended-consequences/

[165] Pancrelipase, Medline Plus, 22 June 2022, https://medlineplus.gov/druginfo/meds/a604035.html

[166] Dexamethasone, MedlinePlus, 20 June 2022, https://medlineplus.gov/druginfo/meds/a682792.html

[167] Prochlorperazine, MedlinePlus, 20 June 2022, https://medlineplus.gov/druginfo/meds/a682116.html

[168] Senna, MedlinePlus, 20 June 2022, https://medlineplus.gov/druginfo/natural/652.html

[169] Stool softeners, MedlinePlus, 20 June 2022, https://medlineplus.gov/druginfo/meds/a601113.html#brand-name-1

[170] Esomeprazole, MedlinePlus, 20 June 2022, https://medlineplus.gov/druginfo/meds/a699054.html#brand-name-1

[171] Hydromorphone, MedlinePlus, 20 June 2022, https://medlineplus.gov/druginfo/meds/a682013.html#brand-name-1

[172] Pegfilgrastim-bmez, Mayo Clinic, 20 June 2022, https://www.mayoclinic.org/drugs-supplements/pegfilgrastim-bmez-subcutaneous-route/description/drg-20476962

[173] Pegfilgrastim-bmez is used to reduce the risk of infection while you are being treated with cancer medicines by stimulating the production of specific WBC's.

[174] Chemotherapy-Induced Diarrhea, Elizabeth A. Koselke, PharmD, Shawna Kraft, PharmD, BCOP, J Hematol Oncol Pharm. 2012;2(4):143-151, https://www.jhoponline.com/jhop-issue-archive/2012-issues/december-2012-vol-3-no-4/15408-chemotherapy-unduced-diarrhea-options

[175] Pantoprazole, Medline Plus, 22 June 2022, https://medlineplus.gov/druginfo/meds/a601246.html

[176] Potassium, R. Morgan Griffin, Melinda Ratini, WebMD, 28 June 2021, https://www.webmd.com/diet/supplement-guide-potassium

[177] Boost Nutritional Drink, 22 June 2022, https://www.boost.com/

178 Boost® Sooth, 22 June 2022, https://www.boost.com/products/boost-soothe#pills-tab

179 Donut hole (Medicare prescription drug), Healthcare.gov, 2 July 2022, https://www.healthcare.gov/glossary/donut-hole-medicare-prescription-drug/

180 High Cost of Pancreatic Enzymes a Barrier for Patients With Cancer, Roxanne Nelson, MedScape, 26 January 2021, https://www.medscape.com/viewarticle/944683?reg=1

181 Morphine Alternatives Compared, Drugs.com, 2 July 2022, https://www.drugs.com/compare/morphine

182 Vital Nutrients Pancreatic Enzymes 1000mg, Amazon, 16 July 2022, https://amzn.to/3Pc8SzW

183 How to Avoid the Medicare Part D Donut Hole, Brandy Bauer, National Council on Ageing (NCOA), 22 Dec 2021, https://www.ncoa.org/article/how-to-avoid-the-medicare-part-d-donut-hole

184 She was already battling cancer. Then she had to fight the bill collectors, Noam Levey, NPR, 9 July 2022, https://www.npr.org/sections/health-shots/2022/07/09/1110370391/cost-cancer-treatment-medical-debt

185 Hitting rewind on the spread of pancreatic cancer, Danielle Ellis, B.Sc., News Medical Life Sciences, 14 July 2022, https://www.news-medical.net/news/20220714/Hitting-rewind-on-the-spread-of-pancreatic-cancer.aspx

186 The Drug Development Process, FDA, 4 January 2018, https://www.fda.gov/patients/learn-about-drug-and-device-approvals/drug-development-process

187 Side Effects in Clinical Trials, DIPG.org, 23 July 2022, https://www.dipg.org/dipg-research/clinical-trials-for-dipg/side-effects/

188 10 dangerous drugs recalled by the FDA, Naveed Saleh, MD, MS, MDLinx, 25 March 2020, https://www.mdlinx.com/article/10-dangerous-drugs-recalled-by-the-fda/lfc-4008

189 What Is Informed Consent?, American Cancer Society, 13 May 2019, https://www.cancer.org/treatment/treatments-and-side-effects/planning-managing/informed-consent/what-is-informed-consent.html

190 A Vanitas Still Life with a Skull, a Book and Roses, c.1630, Meisterdrucke, https://bit.ly/3cfRxrk

191 NY/NJ Trail Conference website, 6 July 2022, https://www.nynjtc.org/

192 New Jersey Search and Rescue website, 6 July 2022, https://www.njsar.org/

193 University of North Carolina, Greensboro I-Corps™ Program, 2 July 2022, https://icorps.uncg.edu/